INTERMITTENT FASTING 16/8

COOKBOOK

The 16:8 Method Step By Step To Lose Weight, Eat Healthy And Feel Better Following This Lifestyle: Includes 50 Delicious Recipes For Breakfast, Lunch, Dinner, And Dessert

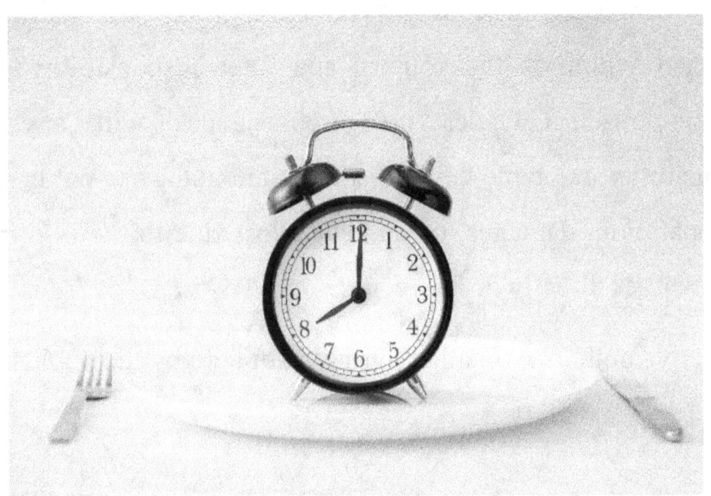

© **Copyright 2020 by Ella Woodridge. All rights reserved.**

In no way is it legal to reproduce, duplicate, or transmit any part of this document in either electronic means or in printed format. Recording of this publication is strictly prohibited and any storage of this document is not allowed unless with written permission from the publisher. All rights reserved.

The information provided herein is stated to be truthful and consistent, in that any liability, in terms of inattention or otherwise, by any usage or abuse of any policies, processes, or directions contained within is the solitary and utter responsibility of the recipient reader. Under no circumstances will any legal responsibility or blame be held against the author or publisher for any reparation, damages, or monetary loss due to the information herein, either directly or indirectly.

Respective authors own all copyrights not held by the publisher.

Legal Notice

This book is copyright protected. This is only for personal use. You cannot amend, distribute, sell, use, quote or paraphrase any part or the content within this book without the consent of the author or copyright owner. Legal action will be pursued if this is breached.

Disclaimer Notice

Please note the information contained within this document is for educational and entertainment purposes only. Every attempt has been made to provide accurate, up to date, and reliable complete information. No warranties of any kind are expressed or implied. Readers acknowledge that the author is not engaging in the rendering of legal, financial, medical or professional advice.

By reading this document, the reader agrees that under no circumstances are the author or publisher responsible for any losses, direct or indirect, which are incurred as a result of the use of information contained within this document, including, but not limited to errors, omissions, or inaccuracies.

Trademarks

The trademarks that are used are without any consent, and the publication of the trademark is without permission or backing by the trademark owner. All trademarks and brands within this book are for clarification purposes only, and are owned by the owners themselves, who are not affiliated with this document.

TABLE OF CONTENTS

WHAT YOU NEED TO KNOW ABOUT INTERMITTENT FASTING AND 16/8

I wrote this book because of the immense success that I've been having with intermittent fasting with my clients who are seeking to lose weight and live healthier. Some are overweight, without any complications, but others have diabetes and non-alcoholic fatty liver disease (NAFLD/NASH) and have been advised to lose weight to help them treat these conditions.

What is Intermittent Fasting?

Intermittent fasting is a feeding pattern that alternates between periods of fasting and controlled eating. It is a simple dietary method divided into many types. One of the methods is alternate day fasting, whereby a person takes a normal diet on particular days of the week and fasts on some. During the fasting days, one does not fully abstain from food but rather reduces calorie intake to a quarter of the normal diet.

The 16/8 Method

The most well tolerated fasting method is where eating is restricted to a certain time window within a day. This means **restricting eating to within an 8 hour window**. This is called the

"16/8 (16:8) Method" – 16 hours of *fasting* and 8 hours of *eating*.

That is what we recommend in this book, since it has worked well for my clients who wish to lose weight. Some people, however, reduce the span to either six, four or even two hours according to their convenience.

How to Implement the 16/8 Method in Your Life

16/8 intermittent fasting is simple, safe and sustainable. To get started, choose an eight-hour window and limit your food intake to that time window.

Most people prefer to eat between 12 p.m. (noon) and 8 p.m. This means that you will only need to fast overnight, and miss breakfast the following morning However, you can still eat a balanced lunch and dinner, along with a few snacks throughout the day. For the snacks, we suggest eating some of the recipes in the Dessert section, or choosing a small savoury item from one of the other sections.

Others opt to eat between 9 a.m. and 5 p.m. This allows you to have a healthy breakfast around 9 a.m., a normal lunch around 12 p.m. (noon), and a light early dinner, or snack, around 4 p.m. before starting your fast.

I suggest that you experiment with the timings, and pick the time span that best fits your daily schedule and preferences. Regardless of when you eat, we recommended that you eat several small meals and snacks spaced evenly through the day. This will help to stabilize blood sugar levels and keep your hunger at bay.

What Types of Food are Good for Intermittent Fasting?

To exploit the potential health benefits of an intermittent fast, it's important to stick to nutritious whole foods and beverages during your eating periods. We recommend balancing each meal with a good variety of healthy whole foods, such as:

- **Good sources of protein:** Meat, poultry, fish, legumes, eggs, nuts, seeds, etc.

- **Veggies:** Broccoli, cauliflower, cucumbers, leafy greens, tomatoes, etc.

- **Whole grains:** Quinoa, rice, oats, barley, buckwheat, etc.

- **Fruits:** Apples, bananas, berries, oranges, peaches, pears, etc.

- **Healthy fats:** Olive oil, avocados and coconut oil etc.

Drinking calorie-free beverages (e.g. water and unsweetened tea and coffee) even while fasting, can also help control your appetite at the same time as keeping you well hydrated.

The recipes in this book have been optimised to include as many of the above ingredients as possible, and to minimize the number of calories in each meal. Overall, this will push you towards losing weight, as long as you stick to eating the recommended number of calories per day or less. For weight loss, a woman should aim to eat approx. 1500 calories per day, whereas a man should try to eat approx. 2000. Studies have shown that this can produce weight loss at a healthy rate (approx. one pound per week). If you find that you are rapidly losing weight on an intermittent fasting diet, then increase the number of calories you are consuming per day until you reach the recommended daily intake (for men 2500 calories; for womean 2000 calories per day).

Health Benefits of Intermittent Fasting

If practiced accordingly, it can result in several positive health benefits. Numerous studies have shown the benefits of intermittent fasting include:

1. *Promoting general body health.* It significantly reduces cravings for snack foods and sugars. The practice normalizes insulin as well as leptin sensitivity. Insulin resistance contributes to many chronic diseases such as diabetes, cancer and heart diseases. Intermittent fasting helps to protect against those diseases.

2. Promoting improved brain health. Fasting helps the body to convert stored glycogen into glucose to release energy. If the fasting proceeds for some time, the continued breakdown of body fats induces the liver to secrete ketone bodies. These small molecules are by-products of fatty acids synthesis, and the brain uses them as fuel. Research also indicates that exercise and fasting

results in genes and other growth factors that are essential in recycling and rejuvenating the brain.

3. *Boosting weight loss.* Combined fasting and exercise increase the effects of catalysts and cellular factors so that the breakdown of glycogen and fats is maximized. Exercising while hungry therefore forces the body to burn stored fats for significant weight loss.

How to take care of yourself

There are a couple of things to note when following an intermittent fasting regime. The most common risk of intermittent fasting is **dehydration**. It is very important you don't forget to drink on the days you do not eat. **Water is essential and black coffee is often used if you get bored with plain water.**

With no food going in the stomach you are **at risk from heartburn** from stomach acid and long-term ulcers that can occur if stomach acid builds up against the stomach walls.

The mental side of fasting also has to be considered. If you fast 2 days a week **don't overindulge** on the other 5, keep to normal meals or it could lead someone to psychological disorders such as bulimia. You also need to be sure you are eating the right **nutrients and minerals**.

Continue to eat fruit and vegetables. If you don't eat for 2 days, make sure the other 5 you are eating enough fruit and vegetables.

Keto/Low–Carb Recipes For Intermittent Fasting

Keto/Low carb diets means limiting carbs to 100 or even 50 grams per day. This means cutting away sugars, starches, and all high carb foods.

Intermittent fasting as said earlier means fasting for a determined period of time. This means your body has to scavenge around for food (fuel), and in the process get rid of damaged cells and other waste that has built up in your body.

Combine the two of these; Low Carb diet & Intermittent Fasting, and you'll have a winning combination to losing weight and feeling great!

We really hope that you love these recipes as much as we do. They are designed to help you lose weight and keep it off by leveraging your natural physiology.

We wish you the best of luck in reaching your body goals!

1.   BREAKFAST RECIPES

Baked Egg In Avocado

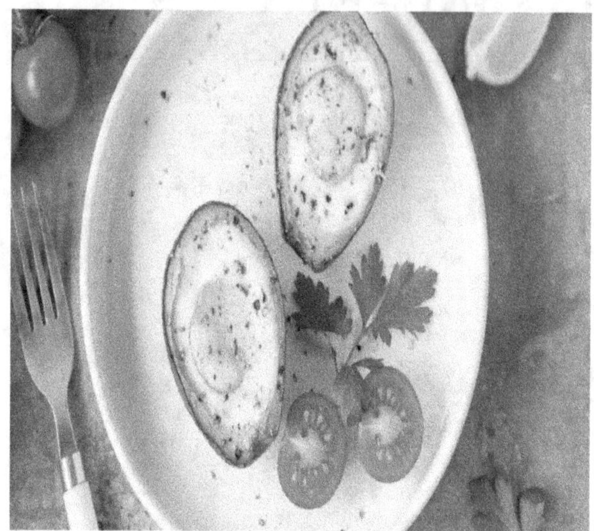

Total Time: 17 Minutes

Servings: 2

Ingredients

- 1 avocado

- 2 egg yolks

- 2 teaspoons olive oil or coconut oil

- Salt and pepper and other seasoning/spices/herbs to taste (smoked paprika goes well with eggs)

Instructions

1. Preheat oven to 400 F (200 C).

2. Slice the avocado in half and remove the stone.

3. Crack the 2 eggs into a bowl.

4. Scoop out each egg yolk and place each into an avocado half.

5. Pour 1 teaspoon of olive oil onto each egg yolk in the avocado.

6. Bake for 12 minutes.

7. Sprinkle salt and pepper and whatever additional herbs and spices you'd like on top.

Nutrition

- Calories: 250 Kcal

- Fat: 23g

- Carbohydrates: 9g

- Protein: 3g

Low-Carb Stack Recipe

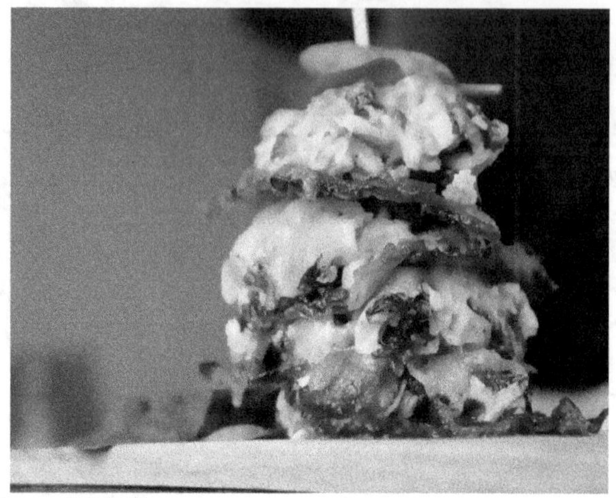

Total Time: 30 Minutes

Servings: 2

Ingredients

- 4 slices bacon (use AIP-compliant bacon if you're staying AIP)

- 1/4 lb (110 g) ground pork

- 1/4 lb (110 g) ground chicken

- 2 teaspoons (2 g) Italian seasoning

- 1 egg, whisked (omit for AIP)

- 1 teaspoon (5 g) salt

- 1/4 teaspoon black pepper (omit for AIP)

- 2 large flat mushrooms (like portobello)

- 1 avocado, sliced

Instructions

1. Cook the bacon until crispy. Leave the fat in the pan.

2. Mix together the ground pork, chicken, Italian seasoning, egg, salt, and pepper in a bowl and form 4 thin patties.

3. Pan-fry the patties in the bacon fat.

4. Then pan-fry the mushrooms.

5. Put together your keto breakfast stack with the mushrooms on the bottom, then 2 thin patties, then 3 slices of avocado, and top it with the slices of bacon. Serve with the rest of the avocado slices.

Nutrition

- Calories: 680 Kcal

- Fat: 54g

- Carbohydrates: 13g

- Protein: 38g

Chicken & Bacon Sausages

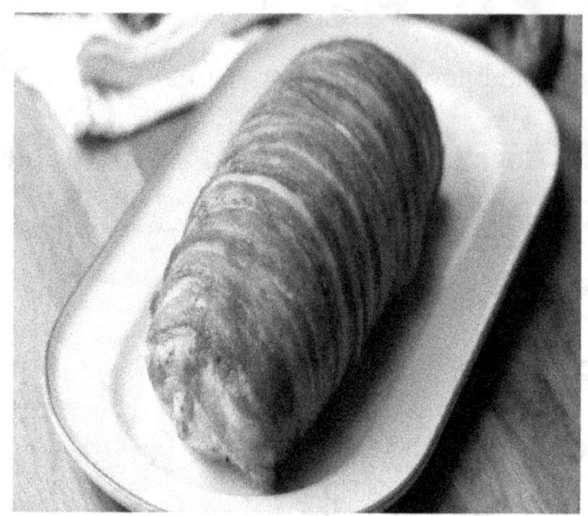

Total Time: 30 Minutes

Servings: 12

Ingredients

- 2 large chicken breasts, or use 1 lb ground chicken

- 2 slices bacon, cooked and broken into small bits

- 1 egg, whisked (omit for AIP)

- 2 Tablespoons Italian seasoning

- 2 teaspoons garlic powder

- 2 teaspoons onion powder

- Salt and pepper

Instructions

1. In a large skillet, melt the coconut oil over medium-high heat. Add the turkey and bacon to the skillet and sauté until slightly browned about 5 to 7 minutes.

2. Add the onion, asparagus, spinach and fresh thyme to the skillet. Sauté for an additional 10 minutes until the turkey and bacon are cooked through and the vegetables are soft.

3. Season with salt and pepper, to taste. .

Nutrition

- Calories: 370 Kcal
- Fat: 21g
- Carbohydrates: 3g
- Protein: 40g

Cinnamon Muffins

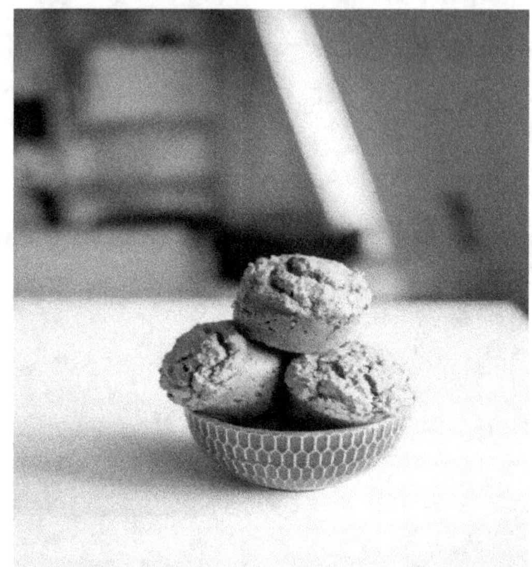

Total Time: 30 Minutes

Yield: 12 Muffins

Ingredients

- 3 cups (180 g) almond flour

- 1/2 cup (120 ml) ghee, melted

- 3 large eggs, whisked

- 3 Tablespoons cinnamon

- 1 teaspoon nutmeg

- 1/4 teaspoon cloves

- 4 Tablespoons (60 ml) applesauce

- 1 teaspoon (5 ml) lemon juice

- Stevia, to taste

- 1 teaspoon baking soda

Instructions

1. Preheat oven to 350 F (175 C).

2. Mix together all the ingredients in a large mixing bowl.

3. Pour into muffin pans (use silicone muffin pans or grease the metal pans). Makes 12 muffins.

4. Bake for 18-20 minutes until a toothpick comes out clean when you insert it into a muffin. .

Nutrition

- Calories: 241 Kcal

- Fat: 22g

- Carbohydrates: 7g

- Protein: 7g

Almond Flour Pancakes

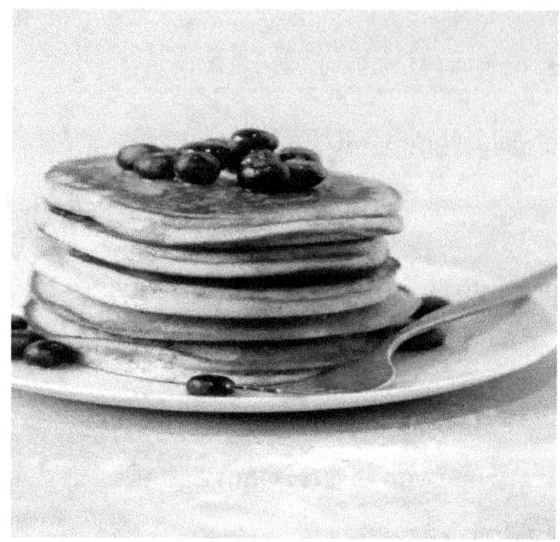

Total Time 20 mins

Servings: 6

Ingredients

- 1 cup blanched almond flour

- 2 eggs

- 2 tablespoons maple syrup (optional; or use water)

- 2 tablespoons olive oil (or any other liquid oil)

- 1 teaspoon baking powder

- 1 teaspoon vanilla extract

- 1/4 teaspoon fine sea salt

Instructions

Skillet Pancakes

1. Preheat a skillet over medium-low heat on the stove. As it heats, stir together the almond flour, eggs, maple syrup (if using), olive oil, baking powder, vanilla, and salt in a large bowl. The batter will be a little thicker than traditional pancake batter.

2. Grease the preheated skillet with butter or olive oil, then pour 3 to 4 tablespoons of the batter into the center of the skillet (I use a scant 1/4 cup). Use a spatula to spread the batter out into a round pancake shape, about 1/4 to 1/2-inch thick.

3. Cook until little bubbles start to form around the edges of the pancake, and as soon as the bottom feels sturdy enough to flip (about 3 to 4 minutes of cooking time), use a spatula to flip the pancake and cook the other side, about 2 to 3 more minutes.

4. Repeat with the remaining batter, until all of the pancakes are cooked. I usually get about 6 pancakes from this batch that are roughly 4 to 6 inches in diameter. Even though they are on the smaller side, they are very filling! Serve warm with your favorite toppings.

Oven-Baked Pancakes

1. Prepare the batter as directed above, but instead of using

the stove preheat the oven to 350°F and line a large baking sheet with parchment paper.

2. Pour the prepared batter by a scant 1/4 cup onto the lined baking sheet, and use a spoon or spatula to spread the batter into a round pancake shape until it's 1/4-inch thick. Leave about 1-inch between each pancake, and repeat with the remaining batter until you have roughly 6 pancakes on the pan.

3. Bake at 350°F for 10 minutes. The pancakes should puff up, and you don't need to flip them, as long as they look like they are thoroughly cooked through. I like to flip them over for serving, so the browned side is on top. Serve warm, with your favorite pancake toppings.

Nutrition

- Calories: 193 Kcal

- Fat: 15g

- Carbohydrates: 9g

- Protein: 6g

Mini Frittata

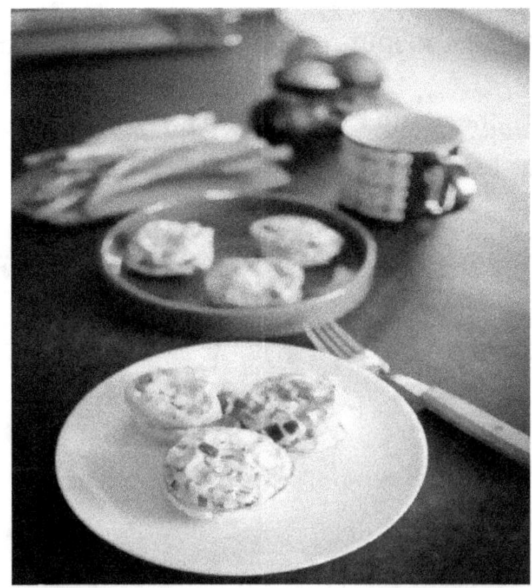

Total Time: 40 Minutes

Yield: 12 Muffins

Ingredients

- 1 cup chopped asparagus (approx. 7–8 spears)

- 4 slices bacon, diced

- 2 Tablespoons chopped onions

- 8 eggs, whisked

- 1/2 cup (120 ml) coconut milk (from can)

- Salt and pepper to taste

Instructions

1. Preheat oven to 350 F (175 C).

2. Cook the diced bacon in a pan.

3. Mix all the chopped vegetables, cooked bacon, whisked eggs and coconut milk together in a large mixing bowl.

4. Pour the batter into muffin cups (makes 12 mini quiches).

5. Bake for 25-30 minutes until the middle of the muffins isn't li□uidy.

Nutrition

- Calories: 460 Kcal

- Fat: 41g

- Carbohydrates: 4g

- Protein: 19g

Avocado With Eggs & Bacon

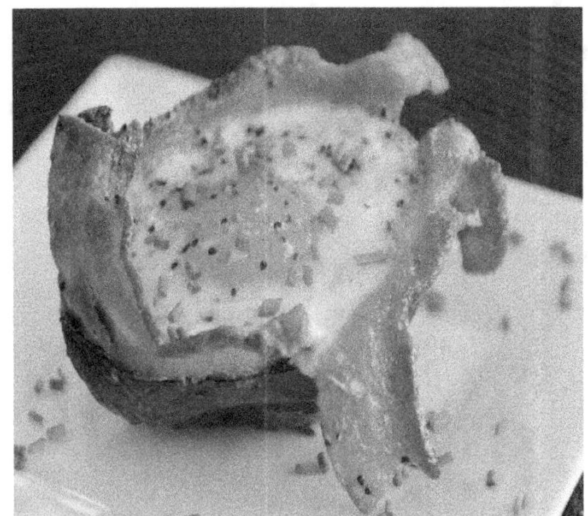

Total Time: 15 min

Servings: 2

Equipment: Airfryer

Ingredients

- 1 ripe avocado

- 2 eggs

- 2 slices bacon, cooked and crumbled

- oil, for spraying

- 1 teaspoon cilantro or parsley, chopped

Instructions

1. Cut avocado in half and remove seed. Scoop out just enough flesh to fit one egg without spilling. Drop one

egg into each avocado half and sprinkle with crumbled bacon.

2. Place avocado halves in air fryer basket and spray with oil. Set the air fryer temperature to 350 degrees, and cook for 5 minutes, or until whites are set and yolks are runny. Sprinkle with cilantro or parsley and serve warm.

Nutrition

- Calories: 362.3 Kcal

- Total Fat: 24.5g

- Net carbs: 2.6g

- Protein: 29.4g

Baked Egg Cups Spinach & Cheese

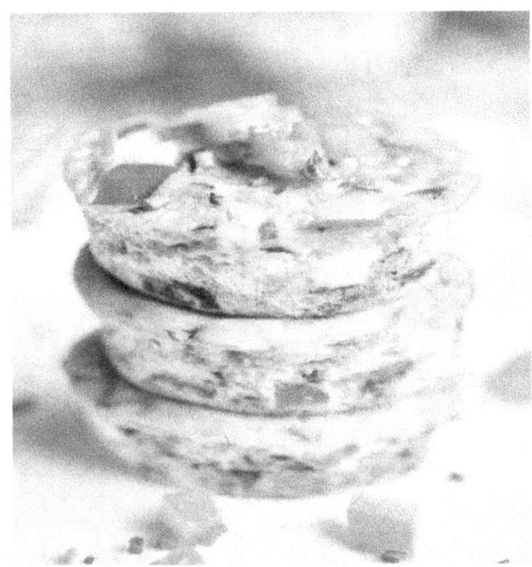

This recipe is written based on one egg, but you can cook as many in a batch that your air fryer will fit without squishing the baking vessels.

If cooking multiple cups at a time, it may take additional time. Or if you're making a 2 eggs in one jumbo sized muffin cup, add an additional 2-4 minutes.

Total Time: 15 mins

Serves: 4

Equipment: Airfryer

Ingredients

- 1 large egg

- 1 tablespoon almond milk or half & half

- 1 tablespoon frozen spinach , thawed (or sautéed fresh

spinach)

- 1-2 teaspoons grated cheese

- salt, to taste

- black pepper, to taste

- Cooking Spray, for muffin cups or ramekins

Instructions

1. Spray inside of silicone muffin cups or ramekin with oil spray.

2. Add egg, milk, spinach and cheese into the muffin cup or ramekin.

3. Season with salt and pepper. Gently stir ingredients into egg whites without breaking the yolk.

4. Air Fry at 330°F for about 6-12 minutes (single egg cups usually take about 6 minutes - multiple or doubled up cups take as much as 12. As you add more egg cups, you will need to add more time.)

5. Cooking in a ceramic ramekin may take a little longer. If you want runny yolks, cook for less time. Keep checking the eggs after 5 minutes to ensure the egg is to your preferred texture.

Nutrition

- Calories: 108 Kcal

- Total Fat: 9g

- Carbohydrates: 2g

- Protein: 8g

Scrambled Eggs

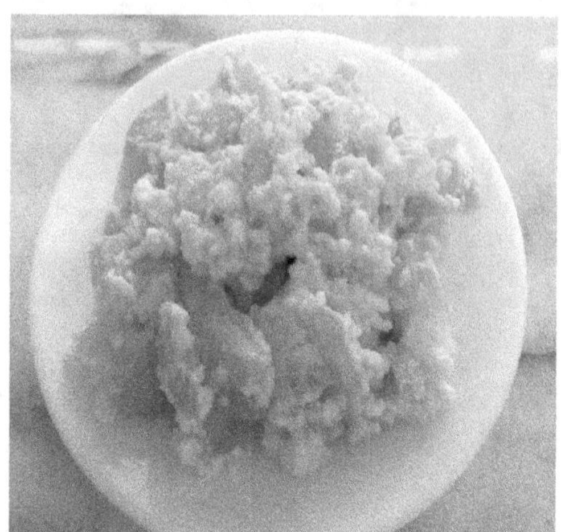

An easy way to make scrambled eggs inside your air fryer to perfection.

Total Time: 12 Min

Serves: 2

Equipment: Airfryer

Ingredients

- 1/3 tablespoon unsalted butter

- 2 eggs

- 2 tablespoons almond milk

- salt and pepper to taste

- 1/8 cup cheddar cheese

Instructions

1. Place butter in an air fryer-safe pan and place inside the air fryer.

2. Cook at 300 degrees until butter is melted, about 2 minutes.

3. Whisk together the eggs and milk, then add salt and pepper to taste.

4. Cook on 300 degrees for 3 minutes, then push eggs to the inside of the pan to stir them around.

5. Cook for 2 more minutes then add cheddar cheese, stirring the eggs again.

6. Cook 2 more minutes.

7. Remove pan from air fryer and enjoy immediately.

Nutrition

- Calories: 126 Kcal

- Total Fat: 9g

- Net Carbohydrates: 1g

- Protein: 9g

Scotch Eggs

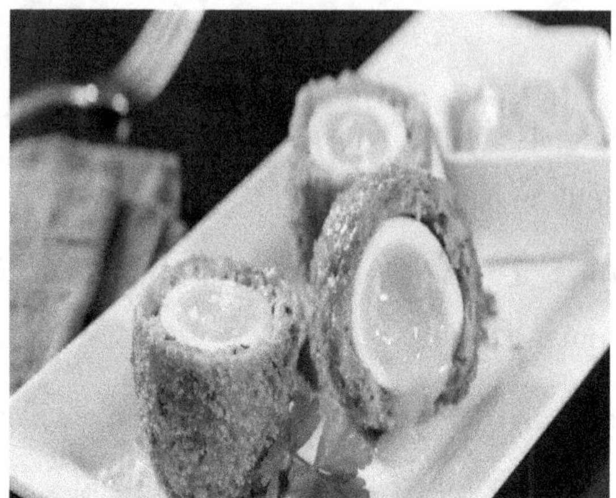

Scotch eggs are the perfect breakfast and brunch dish. It's always a great conversation piece when everyone sees the boiled egg stuffed in sausage. Use whatever your favorite sausage might be: Sweet Italian, Breakfast Sausage, Chicken Apple, etc. Don't forget the swipe of mustard and hot sauce.

Total Time: 30 mins

Servings: 6

Equipment: Airfryer

Ingredients

- 1 pound uncooked bulk sausage

- 5-6 hard boiled eggs

- 1-2 raw eggs , beaten

- 1 cup coating choice (crushed pork rinds, almond flour, coconut flour or preferred coating *see notes below)

- Mustard and/or hot sauce oil spray, for coating

Instructions

1. Peel hard boiled eggs. Divide the sausage into 5 or 6 equal parts, depending on how thick you want the sausage to wrap around the egg.

2. Flatten each portion into a thin patty about 4" wide. Lay boiled egg in center and wrap sausage around the whole egg. Repeat for all eggs.

3. Dip sausage-wrapped egg in beaten raw egg, then in breading. Spray outside of coated egg evenly with oil.

4. Air Fry at 400°F for 12-16 minutes, turn halfway through cooking. The thicker the sausage layer, the longer it takes to cook.

5. Cut in half and serve with mustard swipe on top of yolk. Add hot sauce, too, if you want. Enjoy!!!

Recipe Notes

1. You can add additional flavor to your sausage by mixing it with some Worcestershire, fresh parsley and other spices. If not, simple bulk sausage still tastes great!

2. Coating Choice: If you don't mind a few more carbs, bread crumbs, panko flakes, or crushed crackers work great as breading choices too. For fewer calories, you can omit the coatings (beaten egg & breading). The

sausage-only outside is great, too, but make sure to spray outside of sausage with oil.

Nutrition

- Calories: 323

- Fat: 26g

- Carbohydrates: 1g

- Protein: 20g

Nutrition

Sausage Egg & Cheese Bites

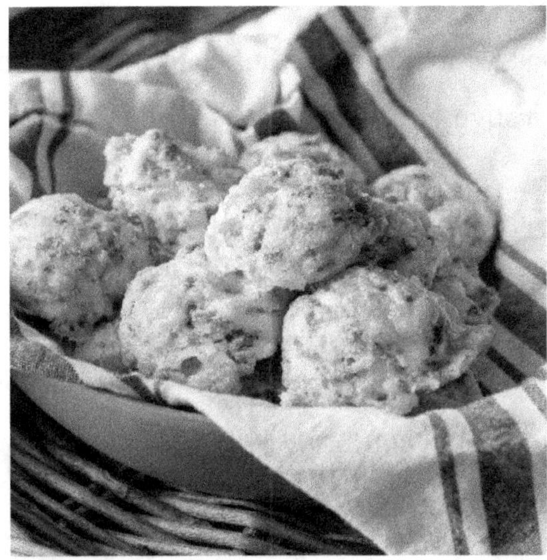

Total Time: 30 min

Serves: 4

Ingredients

- 1 pound breakfast sausage, cooked, drained and cooled slightly

- 4 ounces cream cheese, softened

- 3 eggs, beaten

- 1 cup shredded cheddar

- 1/3 cup coconut flour

- 1/2 teaspoon baking powder

Instructions

1. Preheat oven to 350 degrees.

2. Cook your breakfast sausage, drain and set it aside to cool slightly.

3. When the sausage has cooled add it to a mixing bowl and combine with the cream cheese until there are no cream cheese clumps left.

4. **It is important to make sure the sausage is not too hot before continuing as it will cook the egg when you add it in the next step**

5. Stir in cheese, eggs, coconut flour and baking powder.

6. When the mixture is well incorporated allow it to sit for 5 minutes. Coconut flour continues to absorb moisture so if it seems to runny it won't be.

7. **Skipping this step and not chilling the dough will result in flat bites.

8. Grease a baking sheet and using a small cooking scoop place the Sausage Egg and Cheese Bites on the tray,

Nutrition

- Calories: 79 Kcal

- Carbs: 1.2g

- Proteins: 5g

- Fats: 9g

Ham & Cheese Rolls

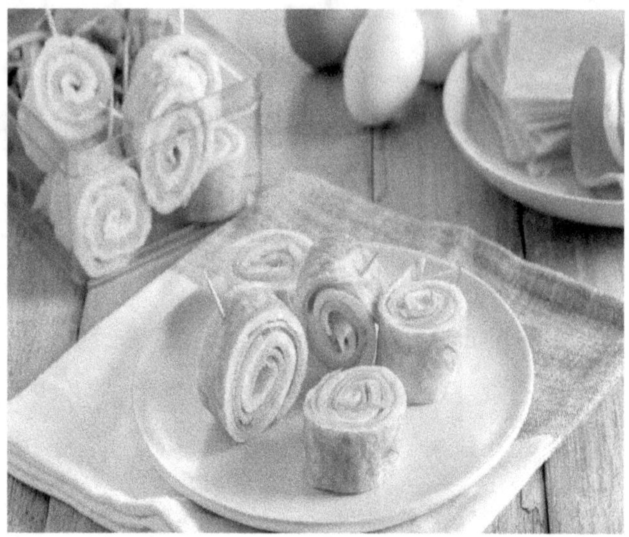

Total time: 20 min

Yield: 6

Ingredients

- 3/4 cup shredded mozzarella cheese.

- 1/2 cup shredded cheddar cheese.

- 1/2 cup grated parmesan , or asiago, other hard, dry, grated cheese.

- 1 cup diced ham

- 2 eggs

Instructions

1. Preheat oven to 375 degrees Fahrenheit.

2. Combine the shredded cheese and egg in a bowl and mix it until the ingredients are fully combined.

3. Stir in diced ham and mix to combine.

4. Set out a well prepped baking sheet - greased or lined with parchment or a silpat.

5. Divide the mixture e☐ually into six to eight parts and form into round rolls.

6. Bake at 375 degrees for about 15 to 20 minutes until the cheese has fully melted and created a slight brown crust.

7. Feel free to mix up your cheese selection - but stick with one grated hard, dry cheese (like parmesan or asiago) to keep the flour-like texture.

Nutrition

- Calories: 198

- Total Fat: 13g

- Carbohydrates: 3g

- Protein: 17g

Arugula, Asparagus & A Poached Egg

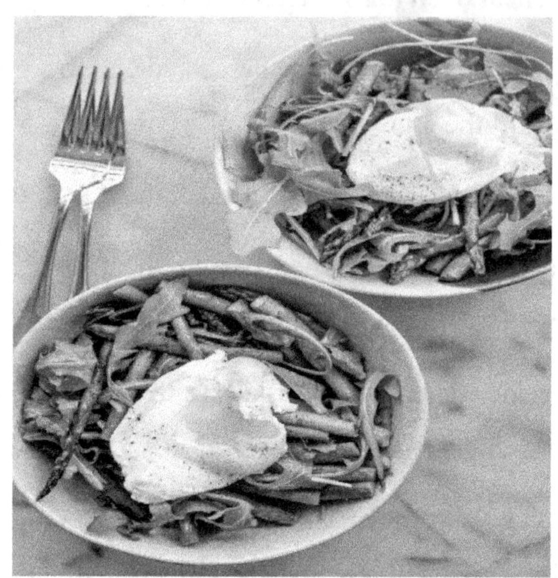

Total Time: 20 Mins

Serves: 2

Ingredients

- dash of white vinegar

- 2 very fresh eggs

- 1 tablespoon olive oil

- 1 bunch asparagus, woody ends removed

- 2 cups arugula

- salt and pepper

- juice of one lemon

Instructions

1. Crack the eggs into individual ramekins or small bowls.

2. Boil at least six cups of water in a large pot, reduce to a heavy simmer and use a spoon to create a whirlpool. Add the vinegar.

3. Drop one egg into the center of the whirlpool and let cook for three minutes. Remove with a slotted spoon and place on a piece of paper towel.

4. Add the second egg to the pot and repeat the process.

5. Meanwhile, in a medium-size frying pan, heat the olive oil over medium high heat.

6. Add the asparagus and cook for at least 6 to 7 minutes or until tender. Use tongs to move it often so all sides of the asparagus are cooked.

7. Add one cup of arugula, half the asparagus, and one egg to each bowl. Sprinkle with salt, pepper, and lemon juice and serve immediately.

Nutrition

- Calories: 172 Kcal
- Fat :12g
- Carbs: 9g
- Protein :11g

Breakfast Pockets

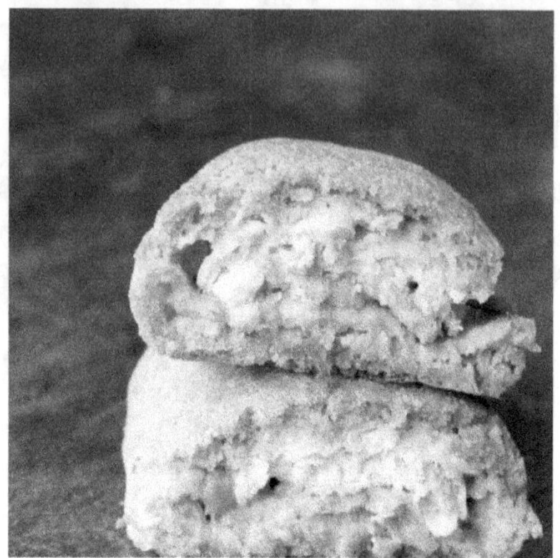

Total Time: 35 mins

Servings: 8

Ingredients:

Dough Ingredients:

- 8 oz mozzarella cheese shredded or cubed

- 2 oz cream cheese

- 2/3 cup almond flour

- 1/3 cup coconut flour

- 1 egg

- 2 tsp baking powder

- 1 tsp salt

Filling Ingredients:

- 2 eggs scrambled

- 4 oz Canadian bacon or other cooked breakfast meat

- 1/2 cup shredded cheddar cheese or other cheese or your choice

Instructions

1. Preheat oven to 350.

2. Put mozzarella cheese and the cream cheese in a microwave-safe bowl. Microwave one minute. Stir. Microwave 30 seconds. Stir. At this point, all the cheese should be melted. Microwave 30 more seconds (it should look like cheese fondue at this point).

3. Put the melted cheese and the other dough ingredients into a food processor and pulse until a uniform dough forms. (Alternatively, you can mix by hand but make sure to knead the dough thoroughly).

4. Divide the dough into 8 pieces. Press each into a 6-inch circle on a piece of parchment paper on a baking sheet. It helps to wet your hands. Divide the filling between each circle of dough. Fold in the edges and crimp to seal. Place back on the parchment seam side down.

5. Bake for 20-25 minutes until golden brown.

Nutrition

- Calories: 258 kcal

- Total Fat: 18g

- Total Carbohydrates: 6g

- Protein: 16g

Airfryer Crispy Chicken Wings

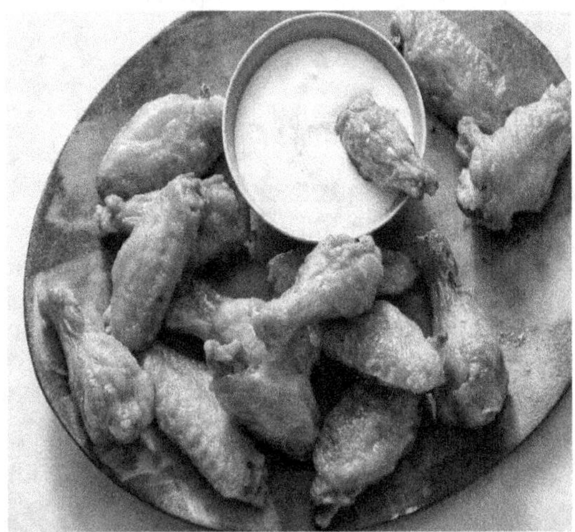

A step-by-step guide for how to cook chicken wings in an air fryer!

Total Time: 40 minutes

Serves: 8

Ingredients

- 2 lb Chicken wings (flats and drumettes, either fresh or thawed from frozen)

- 1 tbsp Gluten-free baking powder

- 3/4 tsp Sea salt

- 1/4 tsp Black pepper

Instructions

1. In a large bowl, toss the wings with baking powder, sea salt and black pepper.

2. Grease 2 racks for the air fryer oven. (If your air fryer only has a basket, grease that instead.)

3. Place the wings onto the greased racks, or place only enough wings into the basket to be in a single layer. (You may need to cook in 2 batches if using a basket.)

4. Place the racks or basket into the air fryer and cook for 15 minutes at 250 degrees.

5. Flip the wings over and switch the trays, so that the top is on the bottom and vice versa. Increase temperature to 430 degrees (or the highest your air fryer goes). Air fry for about 15 to 20 minutes, until chicken wings are done and crispy.

Nutrition

- Calories: 275 Kcal

- Fat: 19g

- Protein: 22g

- Total Carbs: 1g

2.   LUNCH RECIPES

Bacon & Avocado Caesar Salad

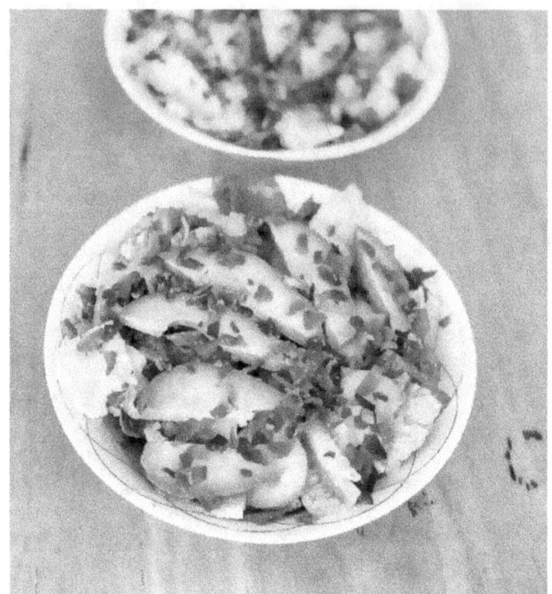

Total Time: 15 Minutes

Servings: 2

Ingredients

For the salad:

- 4 slices of bacon (112 g), diced

- 1 head of romaine lettuce (200 g), chopped

- 1/2 cucumber (110 g), thinly sliced

- 1/4 medium onion (28 g), thinly sliced

- 1 large avocado (200 g), sliced

For the Caesar dressing:

- 1/4 cup of mayo (60 ml)

- 1 Tablespoon of lemon juice (15 ml)

- 1 teaspoon of Dijon mustard (5 ml)

- 1 teaspoon of garlic powder (3.5 g)

- Salt and pepper, to taste

Instructions

1. Add the bacon to a large nonstick skillet over medium-high heat and saute until crispy, about 5 minutes. Remove the bacon from the skillet with a slotted spoon and place on a paper towel-lined plate to cool.

2. In a small bowl, whisk to combine the mayo, lemon juice, mustard, and garlic powder. Season with salt and pepper, to taste.

3. Toss the remaining Caesar dressing with the romaine lettuce leaves. Add the cucumber and onion to the bowl and toss to combine.

Divide the salad between 2 plates and top each salad with equal amounts of cooked bacon and sliced avocado.

Nutrition

- Calories: 652 Kcal

- Fat: 65g

- Carbohydrates: 15g

- Protein: 10g

Salmon with Leek Asparagus

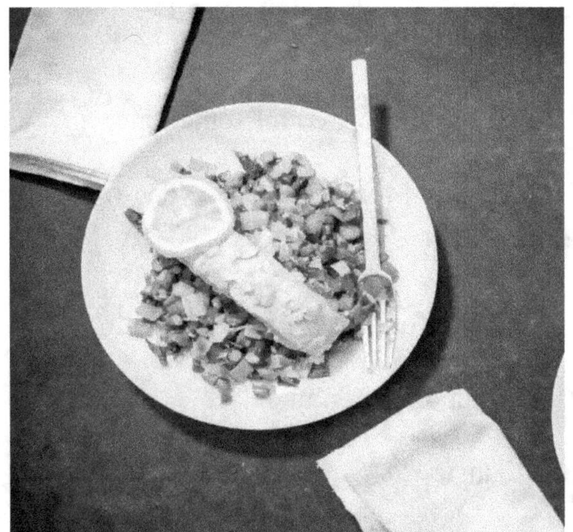

Total Time: 30 Minutes

Servings: 2

Ingredients

For the lemon garlic ghee salmon:

- 2 filets of salmon (with skin on), fresh or frozen (340 g), defrost if frozen

- 1 Tablespoon (15 ml) ghee (use avocado oil for AIP)

- 4 cloves garlic (12 g), minced

- 2 teaspoons (10 ml) lemon juice

- Salt to taste

- Lemon slices, to serve

For the leek asparagus ginger saute:

- 10 spears of asparagus (160 g), chopped into small pieces

- 1 leek (90 g), chopped into small pieces

- 2 teaspoons (4 g) ginger powder (or use finely diced fresh ginger if you have it available)

- Avocado oil or olive oil to saute with

- 1 Tablespoon lemon juice

- Salt to taste

Instructions

1. Preheat oven to 400 F (200 C).

2. Place each salmon filet on a piece of aluminum foil or parchment paper.

3. Divide the ghee, lemon juice, minced garlic between the two filets – place these on top of the salmon. Sprinkle with some salt. Then wrap up the salmon in the foil and place into the oven.

4. Open up the foil after 10 minutes in the oven and then bake for another 10 minutes.

5. While the salmon is cooking, place 1-2 tablespoons of avocado oil or olive oil into a frying pan and saute the chopped asparagus and leek on high heat. Saute for 10

minutes and then add in the ginger powder, lemon juice, and salt to taste. Saute for 1 more minute.

6. Serve by dividing the saute between 2 plates and placing a salmon filet on top of each.

Nutrition

- Calories: 680 Kcal

- Fat: 51g

- Carbohydrates: 15g

- Protein: 4g

Lemon Tuna Salad

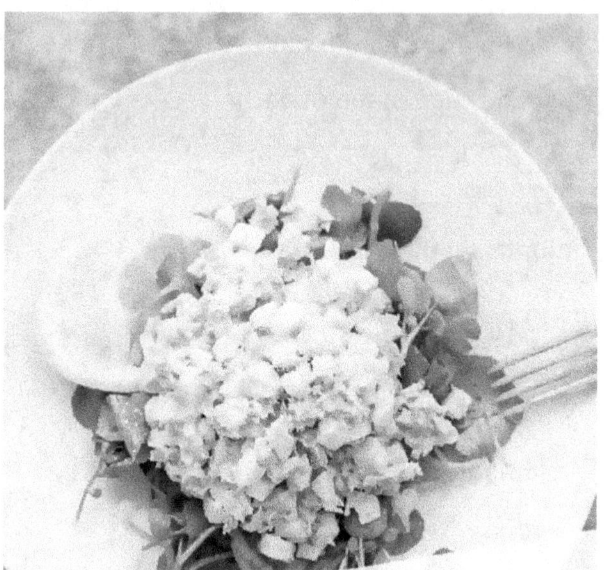

Total Time: 10 Minutes

Servings: 1

Ingredients

- 1/3 cucumber, diced small

- 1/2 small avocado, diced small

- 1 teaspoon lemon juice

- 1 can (4-6 oz or 100–150 g) of tuna

- 1 Tablespoon Paleo mayo (use olive oil for AIP)

- 1 Tablespoon mustard (omit for AIP)

- Salt to taste

- Salad greens (optional)

- Black pepper to taste (omit for AIP)

Instructions

1. Mix together the diced cucumber and avocado with the lemon juice.

2. Flake the tuna and mix well with the mayo and mustard.

3. Add the tuna to the avocado and cucumber. Add salt to taste.

4. Prepare the salad greens (optional: add olive oil and lemon juice to taste).

5. Place the tuna salad on top of the salad greens.

6. Sprinkle black pepper on top.

Nutrition

- Calories: 480 Kcal

- Fat: 40g

- Carbohydrates: 11g

- Protein: 45g

Beef & Broccoli

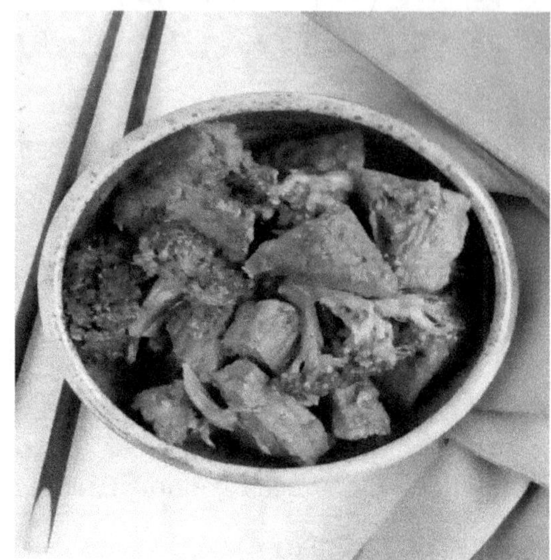

Total Time: 20 Minutes

Servings: 2

Ingredients

- 1 Tablespoon (15 ml) of olive oil

- 14 oz (400 g) of beef sirloin, cut into bite-size pieces

- 1 teaspoon (2 g) of ginger paste (or minced fresh ginger)

- 1 teaspoon (2 g) of garlic paste (or 1 minced garlic clove)

- 1/2 cup (120 ml) of beef broth

- 1 1/2 Tablespoons (23 ml) of gluten-free tamari sauce (or coconut aminos)

- 1/2 head (8 oz or 225 g) of broccoli, broken into small florets

- 1 teaspoon (5 ml) of honey

- Salt and pepper, to taste

Instructions

1. Add the olive oil and beef to the pressure cooker and saute until browned. Add the ginger paste and garlic paste and saute for a few seconds. Add the beef broth, tamari sauce, and broccoli to the pressure cooker, stirring to combine.

2. Secure the lid on the pressure cooker to close. Set the pressure cooker to cook for 10 minutes and then let the pressure release naturally before removing the lid carefully.

3. Remove the beef and broccoli from the pressure cooker with a slotted spoon and set aside to keep warm. To create a sauce, add the honey to the pressure cooker and reduce the liquid by half. Season with salt and pepper, to taste.

4. To serve, place the beef and broccoli on 2 plates and spoon e□ual amounts of the sauce over each plate.

Nutrition

- Calories: 643 Kcal

- Fat: 49g

- Carbohydrates: 10g

- Protein: 37g

Tuscan Chicken Pasta

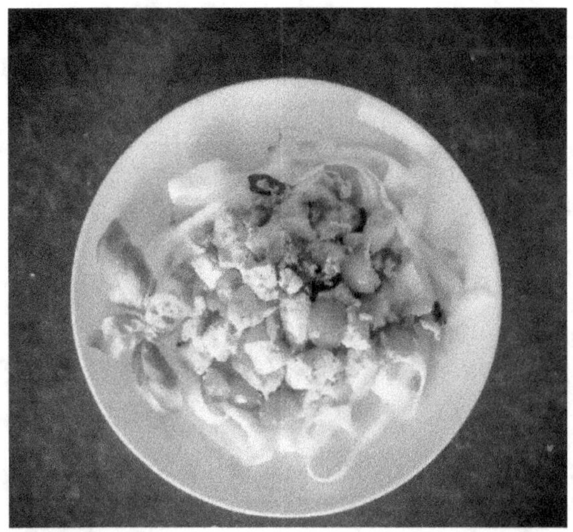

Total Time: 20 Minutes

Servings: 2

Ingredients

- 2 chicken breasts, diced

- 2 small egg, whisked

- 1/4 teaspoon salt

- Dash of black pepper

- 2 teaspoon garlic powder

- 2 teaspoon Italian seasoning

- 14 cherry tomatoes, cut into ⬜uarters

- 30 basil leaves

- Olive oil or avocado oil to cook in

- Additional salt and pepper to taste

- 1 zucchini, peeled and turned into shreds or strands for the pasta

Instructions

1. In a bowl, mix together the whisked egg, salt, pepper, garlic powder, and Italian seasoning.

2. Place the diced chicken pieces into the egg mixture and make sure the chicken is well covered with the mixture.

3. Place 2 tablespoon of olive or avocado oil into a frying pan and saute the chicken pieces coated with the egg mixture until the chicken pieces are fully cooked.

4. Add in the quartered cherry tomatoes and fresh basil leaves. Saute for 2-3 minutes more.

5. Make the zucchini noodles by peeling a zucchini and then using the shredding attachment of a food processor or else using a potato peeler to create pasta-like strands or shreds.

6. Divide the zucchini noodles into two and place onto plates. Top with the sautéed chicken.

Nutrition

- Calories: 540 Kcal

- Fat: 36g

- Carbohydrates: 7g

- Protein: 45g

Garlic Shrimp Caesar Salad

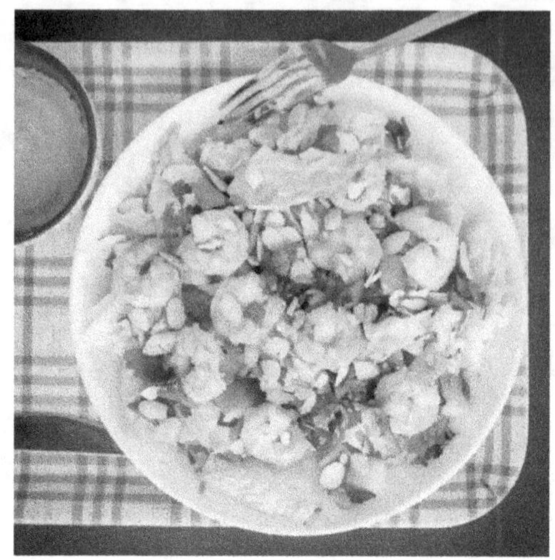

Total Time: 25 Minutes

Servings: 4

Ingredients

For the shrimp:

- 1 lb shrimp (shell removed)

- 2 tablespoons olive oil

- 1 tablespoon lemon juice

- 3 tablespoons garlic powder

- 1 tablespoons onion powder

- Salt and pepper

For the salad:

- 1 head romaine lettuce, chopped

- 1 cucumber, chopped into cubes

For the dressing:

- 1 teaspoon Dijon mustard

- 1/4 cup Paleo mayo (you can purchase this one or make this one)

- 1 tablespoon fresh lemon juice

- 2 teaspoons garlic powder

- Salt and pepper

For garnish:

- 1 tablespoon parsley, chopped

- 1 tablespoon sliced almonds

Instructions

1. Preheat oven to 400F.

2. Mix the shrimp, olive oil, lemon juice, garlic, onion powder, salt and pepper together. Place shrimp on baking tray and roast for 10 minutes.

3. To make the salad dressing, blend the mayo, mustard, lemon juice, garlic powder, salt and pepper together.

4. Toss the dressing with the chopped lettuce, chopped cucumber, and roasted shrimp. Garnish with the

chopped parsley and sliced almonds.

Nutrition

- Calories: 296 Kcal

- Fat: 19g

- Carbohydrates: 7g

- Protein: 25g

Zucchini Noodles With Avocado Sauce

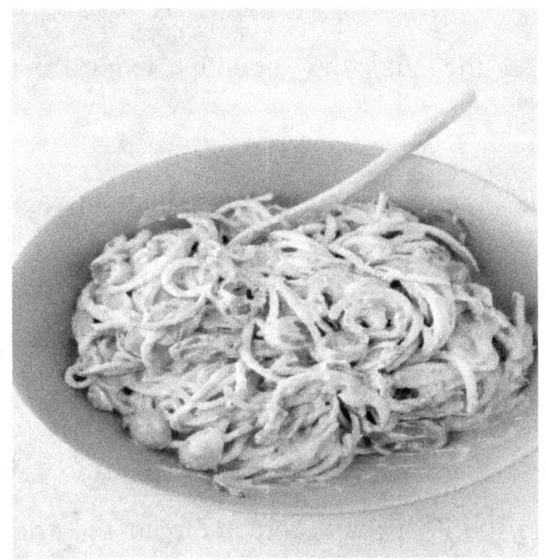

Total time: 10 mins

Servings: 1

These delicious zucchini noodles (or zoodles) with avocado sauce are ready in 10 minutes. Besides, this recipe re□uires just 7 ingredients to make.

Ingredients

- 1 zucchini

- 1 1/4 cup basil (30 g)

- 1/3 cup water (85 ml)

- 4 tbsp pine nuts

- 2 tbsp lemon juice

- 1 avocado

- 12 sliced cherry tomatoes

Instructions

1. Make the zucchini noodles using a peeler or the Spiralizer.

2. Blend the rest of the ingredients (except the cherry tomatoes) in a blender until smooth.

3. Combine noodles, avocado sauce and cherry tomatoes in a mixing bowl.

4. These zucchini noodles with avocado sauce are better fresh, but you can store them in the fridge for 1 to 2 days.

Notes:

- Feel free to use any veggies or fresh herbs you have on hand. You can also spiralize other veggies like carrots, beet, butternut squash, cabbage, etc.

- Any nuts can be used instead of the pine nuts, or even seeds.

Nutrition

- Calories : 313 Kcal

- Fat: 26.8g

- Carbohydrates: 18.7g

- Protein: 6.8g

Chicken Noodle Soup

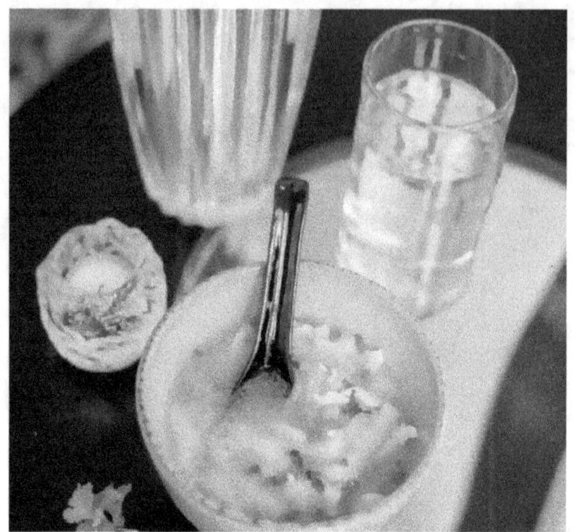

Total Time: 30 Minutes

Yield: 2 bowls

Ingredients

- 3 cups chicken broth (use this recipe or buy this one) (approx 720ml)

- 1 chicken breast, chopped into small pieces (approx 240g or 0.5 lb)

- 2 Tablespoons avocado oil

- 1 stalk of celery, chopped (approx 57g)

- 1 green onion, chopped (approx 10g)

- 1/4 cup cilantro, finely chopped (approx 15g)

- 1 zucchini, peeled (approx 106g)

- Salt to taste

Instructions

1. Dice the chicken breast.

2. Add the avocado oil into a saucepan and saute the diced chicken in there until cooked.

3. Add chicken broth to the same saucepan and simmer.

4. Chop the celery and add it into the saucepan.

5. Chop the green onions and add it into the saucepan.

6. Chop the cilantro and put it aside for the moment.

7. Create zucchini noodles – I used a potato peeler to create long strands, but other options include using a spiralizer or a food processor with the shredding attachment.

8. Add zucchini noodles and cilantro to the pot.

9. Simmer for a few more minutes, add salt to taste, and serve immediately.

Nutrition

- Calories: 310 Kcal

- Fat: 16g

- Carbohydrates: 6g

- Protein: 34g

Delicious Beef Recipe

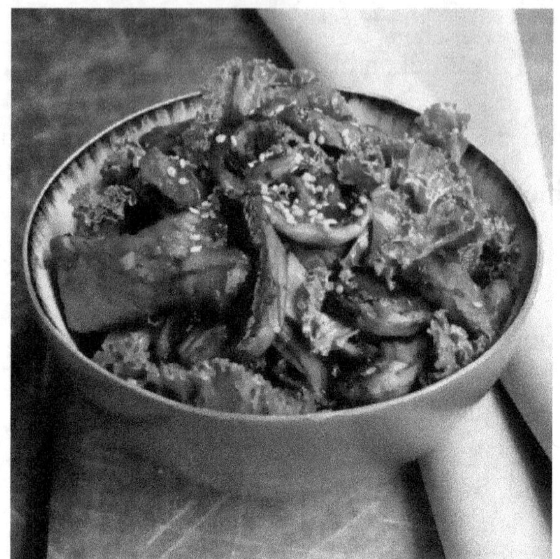

Total Time: 20 Minutes

Servings: 2

Ingredients

- 2 Tablespoons of gluten-free tamari sauce or coconut aminos (30 ml)

- 1 Tablespoon of applesauce (15 ml)

- 2 cloves of garlic (6 g), minced

- 1 Tablespoon of fresh ginger (4 g), minced

- 2 beef sirloin steaks (pick a well marbled steak), sliced

- 1 Tablespoon of sesame seeds (14 g)

- 1 teaspoon of sesame oil

- 2 Tablespoons of avocado oil

- 10 white button mushrooms (100 g), sliced

- 2 oz of curly kale

- Salt and pepper, to taste

Instructions

1. Whisk the tamari sauce, applesauce, garlic and ginger together in a bowl. Add the sliced sirloin and leave to marinate while you prep the remaining ingredients.

2. Toast the sesame seeds in a hot, dry pan until golden. Remove and set aside.

3. Heat the avocado oil in a large wok or frying pan and add the mushrooms, cooking until caramelised. Add the steak slices and the marinade and fry for 2-3 minutes, adding the kale towards the end, stirring into the mixture to gently wilt.

4. Add in the sesame oil and salt and pepper to taste.

5. Serve over cooked cauliflower rice if desired, and top with toasted sesame seeds.

Nutrition

- Calories: 675 Kcal

- Fat: 53g

- Carbohydrates: 9g

- Protein: 38g

Turkey & Vegetable Skillet

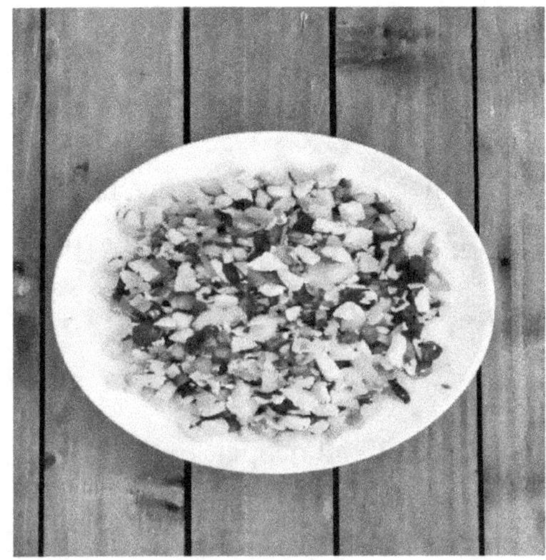

Total Time: 25 Minutes

Servings: 2

Ingredients

- 3 Tablespoons of coconut oil (90 ml), to cook with

- 0.75 lb of turkey breasts (335 g), diced (or ground turkey)

- 4 slices of bacon (112 g), diced

- 1/2 medium onion (55 g), diced

- 3 spears of asparagus (45 g), chopped

- 1 cup of spinach (30 g), chopped

- 4 teaspoons of fresh thyme (4 g), chopped

- Salt and pepper, to taste

Instructions

1. In a large skillet, melt the coconut oil over medium-high heat. Add the turkey and bacon to the skillet and sauté until slightly browned about 5 to 7 minutes.

2. Add the onion, asparagus, spinach and fresh thyme to the skillet. Sauté for an additional 10 minutes until the turkey and bacon are cooked through and the vegetables are soft.

3. Season with salt and pepper, to taste.

Nutrition

- Calories: 665 Kcal

- Fat: 52g

- Carbohydrates: 5 g

- Protein: 47g

Vegan Thai Soup

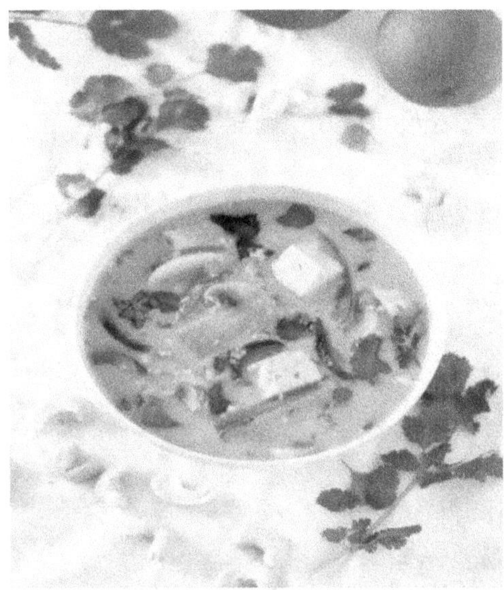

Total Time: 25 Minutes

Serves: 3-4

You only need one pot to make this delicious vegan Thai soup. It's made with easy to get ingredients and you can add your favorite veggies.

Ingredients

- 1/2 julienned red onion
- 1/2 julienned red bell pepper
- 3 sliced mushrooms
- 2 cloves of garlic, finely chopped
- 1/2-inch piece of ginger root (about 1 cm), peeled and

finely chopped

- 1/2 Thai chili, finely chopped* - You can use any chili as well.

- 2 cups vegetable broth or water (500 ml)

- 1 14-ounce can coconut milk (400 ml)

- 1 tbsp coconut, cane or brown sugar

- 10 oz firm tofu, cubed (275 g)

- 1 tbsp tamari or soy sauce

- The juice of half a lime

- A handful of fresh cilantro, chopped

Instructions

1. Place all the veggies (onion, red bell pepper, mushrooms, garlic, ginger and Thai chili), broth, coconut milk and sugar in a large pot.

2. Bring it to a boil and then cook over medium heat for about 5 minutes.

3. Add the tofu and cook for 5 minutes more.

4. Remove from the heat, add the tamari, lime juice and fresh cilantro. Stir and serve.

5. Keep the soup in a sealed container in the fridge for up to 5 days. You can also freeze it.

Nutrition

- Calories: 339 Kcal

- Fat: 27.6g

- Carbohydrates: 15.6 g

- Protein: 14.8 g

Keto Chili

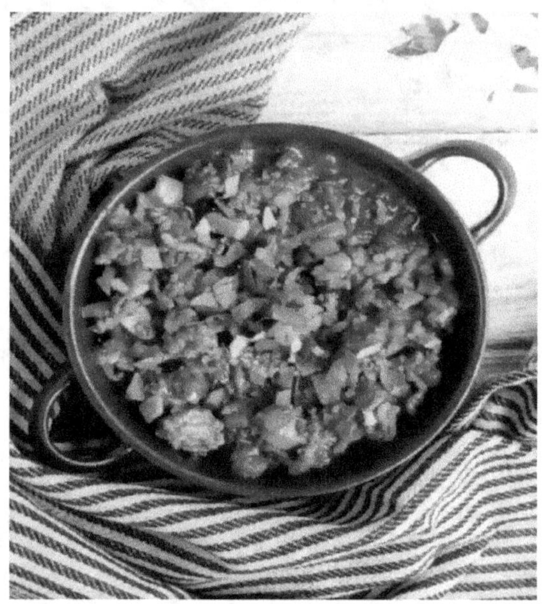

Total time: 40 Minutes

Servings: 6

Ingredients

- 1 pound of lean ground beef

- 2 cloves garlic crushed

- 1 tablespoon olive oil

- 1 medium onion roughly chopped

- 28 oz can crushed tomato

- 1 cup of chopped cherry tomatoes

- 1 cup of water

- 1 ½ teaspoons of sea salt

- 2 tablespoons of chili powder

- ½ tsp ground cayenne pepper

- 1 tablespoon of cumin powder

- 1 teaspoon of garlic powder

- 2 teaspoons of onion powder

Instructions

1. Brown the ground beef, onions, garlic

2. Add the can of tomatoes, fresh tomatoes, water, and spices.

3. Allow to simmer on medium low heat for 30-45 minutes.

4. Alternatively you can cook this chili in slow cooker to do so refer to the notes section.

5. This recipe double and freezes well.

Notes:

Slow Cooker Instructions:

Add all the ingredients into your slow cooker and break up the ground beef and then set to low. Your Keto Chili will be done in 4-6 hours based on your specific slow cooker.

Nutrition

- Calories: 178 Kcal

- Total fat: 5.5g

- Carbohtydrates: 7.3g

- Protein: 24.3g

Zuppa Toscana

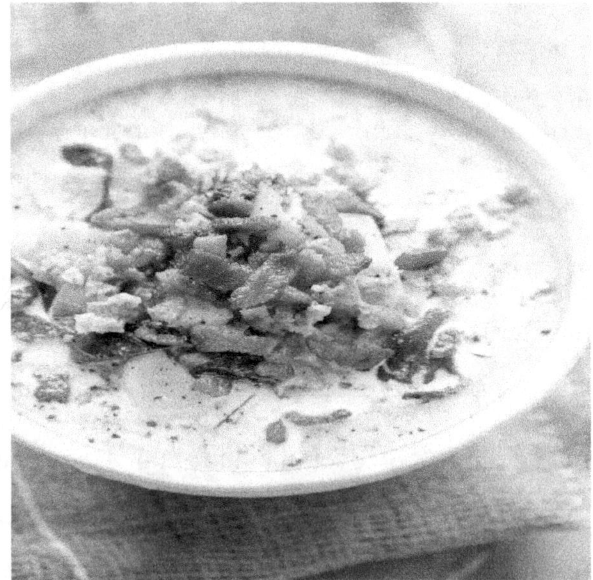

Total Time: 55 minutes

Serves: 8

Ingredients

- 6 slices bacon, roughly chopped

- 1 lb ground mild Italian sausage

- 1 tbsp (14g) butter

- 2 tsp (10g) minced garlic

- ½ tsp ground sage

- ¼ tsp black pepper

- 2 ¾ cups chicken broth

- ¾ cup heavy whipping cream

- ¼ cup shredded parmesan cheese

- 1 lb radishes, quartered

- 2 oz kale, de-stemmed, roughly chopped

Instructions

1. To a large pot over medium heat, cook chopped bacon until crisp. Transfer bacon to a paper-towel-lined plate and dispose of grease, but do not wash the pan.

2. In the same pot over medium-high heat, cook ground sausage until browned, breaking the meat apart with a wooden spoon while cooking. Transfer browned sausage to a paper towel-lined plate and dispose of grease, but do not wash the pan.

3. To same pot over medium heat, melt butter. Add garlic and spices and saute until fragrant, about 1 minute. Increase heat to medium-high and add in chicken broth, heavy cream, and shredded parmesan. Bring mixture to a simmer, add □uartered radishes, and decrease the heat to medium-low. Simmer until radishes are fork-tender, about 15-20 minutes.

4. Stir in browned sausage and chopped kale and continue to simmer until kale wilts, about 5-10 minutes, before serving in bowls. Garnish soup with crisped bacon

crumbles.

Nutrition:

- Calories: 334 Kcal

- Total Fat: 31g

- Total Carbohydrate: 3.9g

- Protein: 12g

Taco Casserole

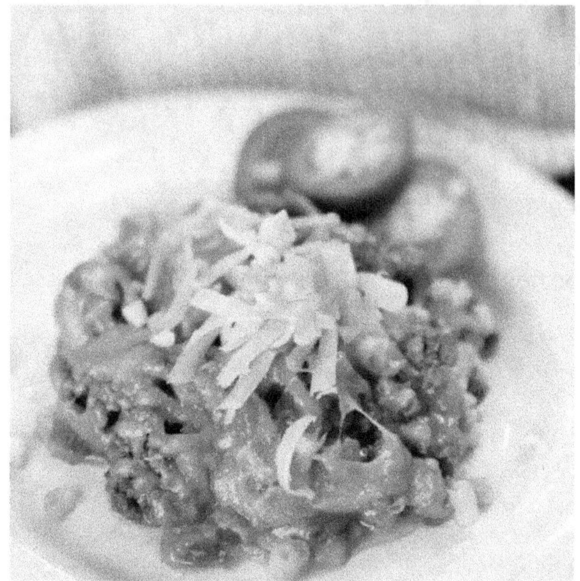

Total Time: 40 min

Serves: 6

Ingredients

- 1 1/2 lb ground beef
- 1 14.5 oz can chopped tomatoes
- 1 4 oz can diced green chiles
- 2 cups cooked cauliflower rice
- 3 Tbs taco seasoning
- 1 8 oz bag taco cheese

Instructions

1. Cook the cauliflower rice (either bagged or fresh) and pat dry to remove excess moisture

2. Cook beef on stovetop until brown

3. Add tomatoes, cauliflower, taco seasoning and chiles and stir until well mixed

4. In a 13 x 9 baking dish, layer enough of the beef mixture to cover the bottom - about half

5. Top with 2/3 of the cheese and spread evenly

6. Repeat with the rest of the beef and then top with the rest of the cheese

7. Bake for 15-20 min at 350 degrees until cheese is melted

8. Serve in a bowl alone or with sour cream and avocado

Nutrition

- Calories: 522 Kcal

- Total Fat: 31g

- Carbohydrates: 10g

- Protein: 42g

3. DINNER RECIPES

Broccoli Bacon Salad & Coconut Cream

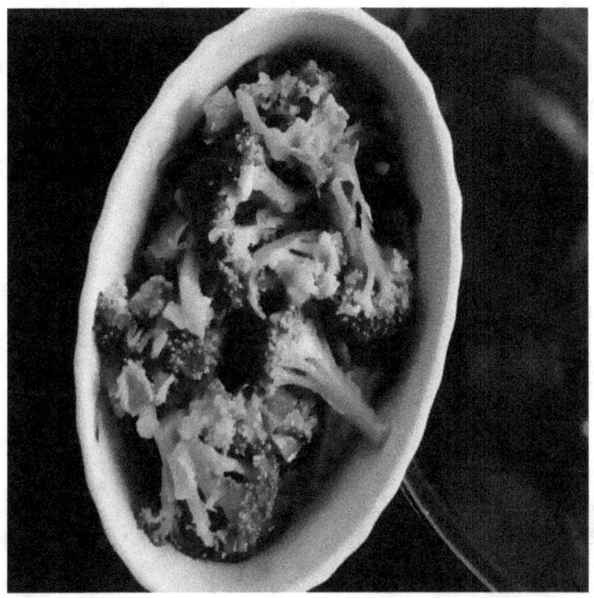

Total Time: 40 Minutes

Servings: 6

Ingredients

- 1 lb broccoli florets

- 4 small red onions or 2 large ones, sliced

- 20 slices of bacon, chopped into small pieces

- 1 cup coconut cream

- salt to taste

Instructions

1. Cook the bacon first, and then cook the onions in the

bacon fat.

2. Blanche the broccoli florets (or you can use them raw or
    have them softer by boiling them).

3. Toss the bacon pieces, onions, and broccoli florets
    together with the coconut cream and salt to taste.

4. Serve at room temperature.

Nutrition

- Calories: 280 Kcal

- Fat: 26g

- Carbohydrates: 8g

- Protein: 7g

Chicken Mushroom Casserole

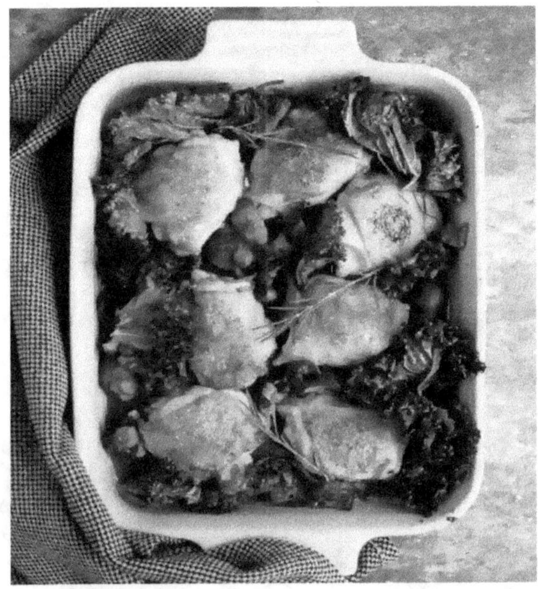

Total Time: 50 Minutes

Servings: 4

Ingredients

- 4 Tablespoons of avocado oil (30 ml), to cook with

- 8 chicken thighs (with skin on) (1.2 kg)

- 1 medium onion (110 g), peeled and thinly sliced

- 3 cloves of garlic (9 g), peeled and chopped

- 2 Tablespoons of fresh rosemary (6 g), chopped

- 30 white button mushrooms (300 g), halved

- 2 oz of kale (56 g)

- Salt and freshly ground black pepper

- Additional rosemary sprigs for garnish (optional)

Instructions

1. Preheat the oven to 350°F (180°C).

2. Add avocado oil to a frying pan and brown the chicken thighs skin-side down until golden and crispy, then turn the thighs over and cook the other side for a minute or two.

3. The chicken isn't cooked right now, but they'll be finished off in the oven. Carefully remove from the frying pan and put into a roasting dish.

4. Using the leftover oil in the pan, cook the sliced onions, garlic and rosemary and cook over a low-moderate heat to soften the onions completely. Turn the heat up and keep cooking the onions for a few more minutes until they become jammy. Add the mushrooms to the frying pan for a few minutes.

5. Spoon the mushrooms and jammy onions into the roasting tray around the chicken pieces and place the dish in the oven for 20 minutes.

6. In the meantime, toss the kale in some more olive oil.

7. After 20 minutes, increase the oven temperature to 400 F (200 C) and remove the tray from the oven while it

heats. Scatter the oiled kale in and around the dish, then return the dish to the oven for an additional 5 minutes.

8. Season with salt and freshly ground black pepper, as well as additional rosemary sprigs, then serve to the table for everyone to help themselves.

Nutrition

- Calories: 553 Kcal

- Fat: 42g

- Carbohydrates: 7g

- Protein: 35g

Creamy Salmon Pasta

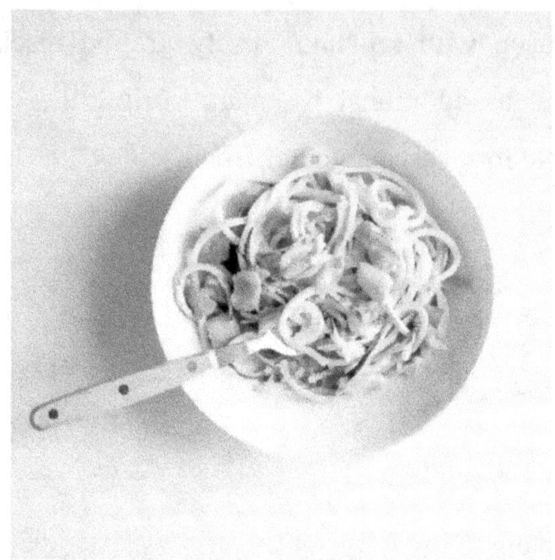

Total Time: 10 Minutes

Servings: 2

Ingredients

- 2 Tablespoons of coconut oil (30 ml), to cook with

- 8 oz of smoked salmon (224 g), diced

- 2 zucchinis (240 g), spiraled or use a peeler to make into long noodle-like strands

- 1/4 cup of mayo (60 ml)

Instructions

1. In a skillet, melt the coconut oil over medium-high heat. Add the smoked salmon and sauté until slightly browned, about 2 to 3 minutes.

2. Add the zucchini "noodles" to the skillet and sauté until soft, about 1 to 2 minutes.

3. Add the mayo to the skillet, stirring well to combine.

4. Divide the "pasta" between 2 plates and serve.

Nutrition

- Calories: 470 Kcal

- Fat: 42g

- Carbohydrates: 4g

- Protein: 21g

Salmon Cakes

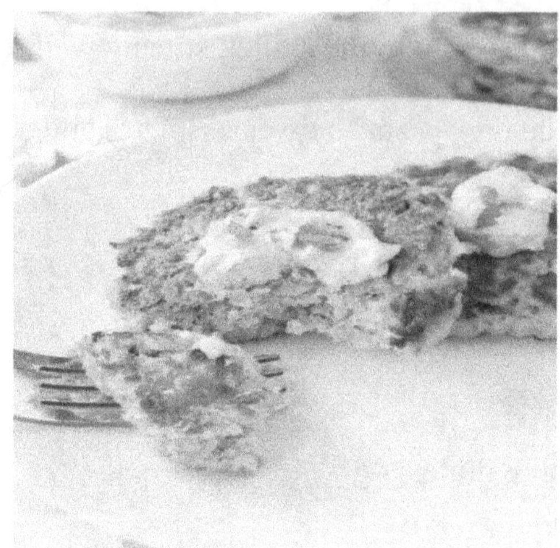

Total time: 12 min

Servings: 2

Ingredients

- Two 5 oz pouch of pink salmon (or cans, drained well)

- 1 egg

- 1/4 cup finely ground pork rinds (optional, but helps)

- 1/2 jalapeno, finely chopped

- 2 tbsp sarayo (or plain mayo)

- 2 tbsp finely diced red onion

- 1/4 tsp garlic powder

- 1/4 tsp chili powder

- Salt and pepper to taste

- 1 tbsp avocado oil

- avocado cream sauce

- 1 avocado

- 1/4 cup sour cream

- 3 tbsp cilantro

- 1–2 tbsp avocado oil (to thin)

- 1–2 tsp Water, to desired thickness

- Juice of half lemon

- Salt, pepper to taste

Instructions

1. In large bowl mix salmon, egg, jalapeno, sarayo, red onion, ground pork rinds and seasoning

2. Form patties with mixture (4 large or 5-6 small)

3. In non stick skillet, drizzle oil and cook patties over medium heat 4-5 minutes until each side is golden brown and crispy

4. avocado sauce

5. Blend all ingredients in food processor until smooth

6. Serve salmon cakes hot with avocado sauce and extra drizzle of sarayo

Nutrition

- Calories: 542 Kcal
- Fat: 50g
- Carbohydrates: 10g
- Protein: 10g

Cobb Egg Salad

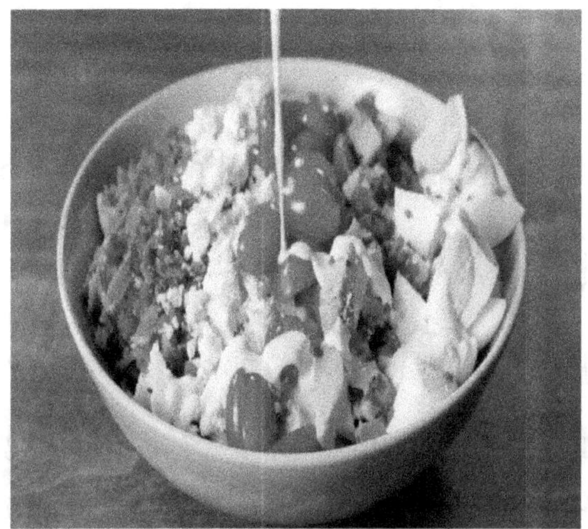

Total Time: 15 min

Serves: 2

Ingredients

- 3 tablespoons nonfat plain yogurt

- 3 tablespoons low-fat mayonnaise

- ¼ teaspoon garlic powder

- ¼ teaspoon freshly ground pepper

- ⅛ teaspoon salt

- 8 hard-boiled eggs

- 1 ripe avocado, cubed

- 2 slices bacon, cooked and crumbled

- ¼ cup crumbled blue cheese

Instructions

1. Combine yogurt, mayonnaise, garlic powder, pepper and salt in a medium bowl. Halve eggs and discard 4 of the yolks (or save for another use). Add whites and the remaining 4 yolks to the bowl and mash to desired consistency. Gently stir in avocado, bacon and blue cheese.

2. Make Ahead Tip: Cover and refrigerate for up to 2 days.

3. Tip: To hard-boil eggs, place eggs in a single layer in a saucepan; cover with water. Bring to a simmer over medium-high heat. Reduce heat to low and cook at the barest simmer for 10 minutes. Remove from heat, pour out hot water and cover the eggs with ice-cold water. Let stand until cool enough to handle before peeling.

Nutrition

- Calories: 235 Kcal

- Fat: 17g

- Carbohydrates: 3g

- Protein: 13g

Crack Chicken Recipe

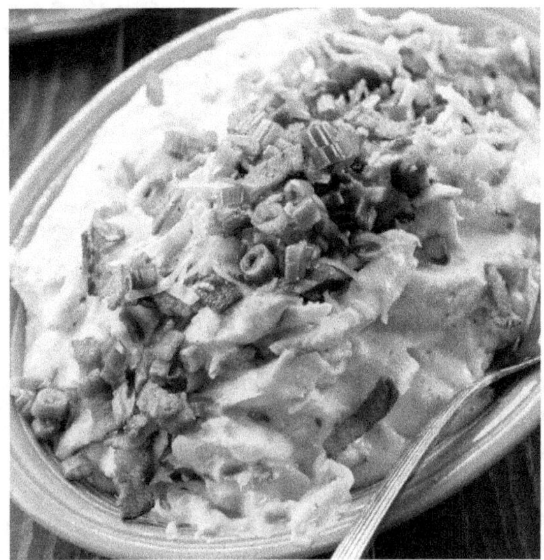

Total Time: 25 minutes

Servings: 8

E☐uipment

- pressure cooker

Ingredients

- 2 slices bacon chopped

- 2 lbs boneless skinless chicken breasts

- 16 oz cream cheese

- 1/2 cup water

- 2 tablespoons apple cider vinegar

- 1 tablespoon dried chives

- 1 1/2 teaspoons garlic powder

- 1 1/2 teaspoons onion powder

- 1 teaspoon crushed red pepper flakes

- 1 teaspoon dried dill

- 1/4 teaspoon salt

- 1/4 teaspoon black pepper

- 1/2 cup shredded cheddar (2 oz)

- 1 scallion green and white parts, thinly sliced

Instructions

1. Turn pressure cooker on, press "Sauté", and wait 2 minutes for the pot to heat up. Add the chopped bacon and cook until crispy. Transfer to a plate and set aside. Press "Cancel" to stop sautéing.

2. Add the chicken, cream cheese, water, vinegar, chives, garlic powder, onion powder, crushed red pepper flakes, dill, salt, and black pepper to the pot. Turn the pot on Manual, High Pressure for 15 minutes and then do a Quick release.

3. Use tongs to transfer the chicken to a large plate, shred it with 2 forks, and return it back to the pot.

4. Stir in the cheddar cheese.

5. Top with the crispy bacon and scallion, and serve.

Nutrition

- Calories: 380 kcal

- Carbohydrates: 4g

- Protein: 30g

- Fat: 27g

Crab Stuffed Mushrooms With Cream Cheese

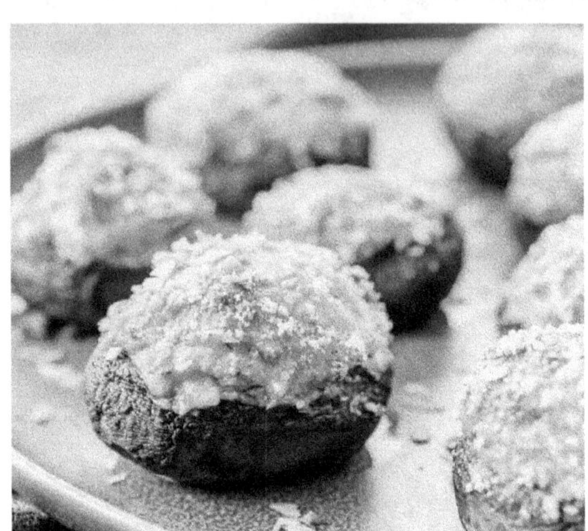

Total Time: 45 minutes

Serves: 4

Ingredients

- 20 ounces cremini (baby bella) mushrooms (20-25 individual mushrooms)

- 2 tablespoons finely grated parmesan cheese

- 1 tablespoon chopped fresh parsley

- salt

Filling:

- 4 ounces cream cheese softened to room temperature

- 4 ounces crab meat finely chopped

- 5 cloves garlic minced

- 1 teaspoon dried oregano

- 1/2 teaspoon paprika

- 1/2 teaspoon black pepper

- 1/4 teaspoon salt

Instructions

1. Preheat the oven to 400 F. Prepare a baking sheet lined with parchment paper.

2. Snap stems from mushrooms, discarding the stems and placing the mushroom caps on the baking sheet 1 inch apart from each other. Season the mushroom caps with salt.

3. In a large mixing bowl, combine all filling ingredients and stir until well-mixed without any lumps of cream cheese. Stuff the mushroom caps with the mixture. Evenly sprinkle parmesan cheese on top of the stuffed mushrooms.

4. Bake at 400 F until the mushrooms are very tender and the stuffing is nicely browned on top, about 30 minutes. Top with parsley and serve while hot.

Nutrition

- Calories: 160 Kcal

- Total Fat: 11g

- Total Carb: 5.5g

- Protein: 9g

Grilled Chicken Salad

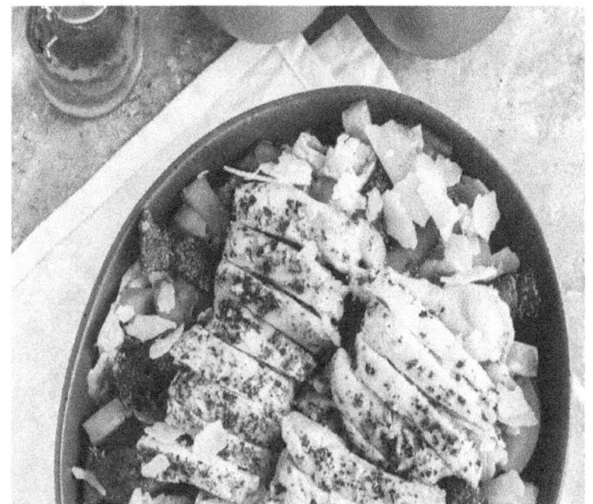

Total Time: 25min

Serves: 2

Ingredients

- 2 Chicken Thighs
- 1 Cup Romain Lettuce
- 1 Slice Bacon
- tsp ½oregano
- 1/2 tsp Salt
- 1/2 tsp Pepper
- 1 tablespoon olive oil
- 2 tablespoons Parmesan cheese

Dressing

- 2 Tablespoons Mayonaise

- 1 tablespoon Dijon Mustard

- 1 teaspoon Lemon Juice

Instructions:

1. Preheat an oven to 180 C (355F) and place the chicken thighs on a baking tray, covered in oregano, olive oil, salt and pepper.

2. Bake the chicken for 15 mins or until cooked right through.

3. You can cook the bacon in the oven if you wish as well, but I prefer cooking it in a frying pan.

4. Heat a frying pan to medium high and place the strip of bacon into the pan. Cook for 5-10 mins until crispy.

5. In a small container or bowl, add together the mayonnaise, Dijon mustard and lemon juice. Mix until combined well.

6. Remove the chicken from the oven, slice into strips. Do the same with the bacon.

7. In your salad bow, add the dressing to your sliced lettuce, and coat the lettuce leaves in as much of the dressing as you can.

8. Add the sliced chicken and bacon, seasoning with parmesan cheese.

Nutrition

- Calories: 187 Kcal

- Fat: 14g

- Carbs: 1g

- Protein: 12g

Chicken Avocado Salad With Sesame Sauce

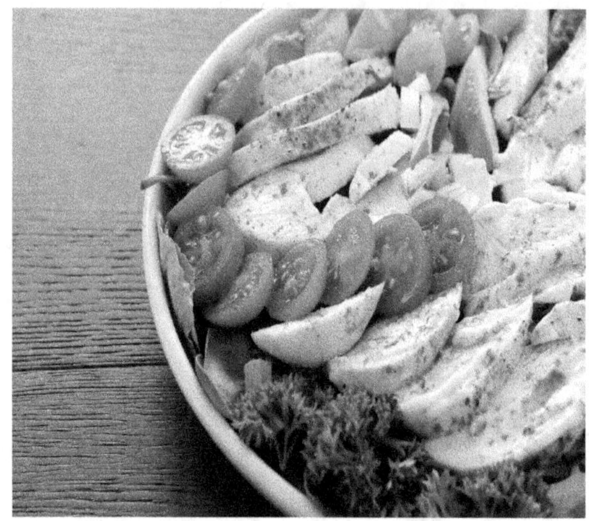

Total Time: 30 minutes

Servings: 1

Ingredients

- 1 Chicken Breast

- 3 Cherry Tomatoes

- 1/2 Avocado

- 1 Tbsp Red Onion

- 2 Tbsp Sesame Seed Oil

- 1 Handful Lettuce

- 2 Tbsp Mayonnaise

- 1 Tsp Paprika, Optional

Instructions

1. Place the chicken breast on a baking tray and cook at 180° C (375° F) for 20 mins (optionally add paprika to the top of the chicken breast at this point)

2. Cut up the salad ingredients to your liking, place on a plate (usually i use the lettuce as a bed to place all the other ingredients on

3. Cut the chicken into pieces and place onto salad. Mix the mayonnaise with the sesame seed oil and use as a dressing.

Nutrition

- Calories: 852

- Fat: 45g

- Carbohydrates: 5g

- Protein: 65g

Crunchy Bacon & Egg Salad

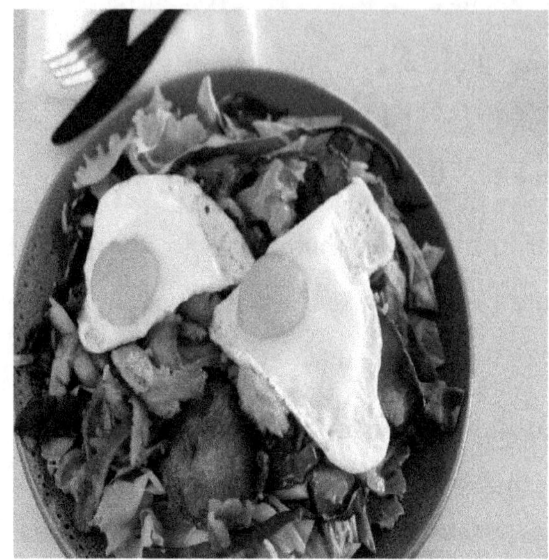

Total Time 15 minutes

Serves: 1

Ingredients

- 2 Eggs

- 2 Slices Bacon (50g / 1.7 oz)

- Handful Lettuce Thinly Sliced

- Handful Red Cabbage Thinly Sliced

Instructions

1. Cook the bacon for about 5-7 mins or until its cooked to the desired consistency,

2. Fry the eggs and keep them sunny side up.

3. Thinly slice the lettuce and red cabbage, line the container or plate with these ingredients, and place the bacon and eggs on top. If you cooked your eggs a little longer, feel free to drizzle some olive oil over the salad.

Nutrition

- Calories: 456 Kcal

- Fat: 32g

- Carbohydrates: 4g

- Protein: 29g

Buffalo Chicken Tenders

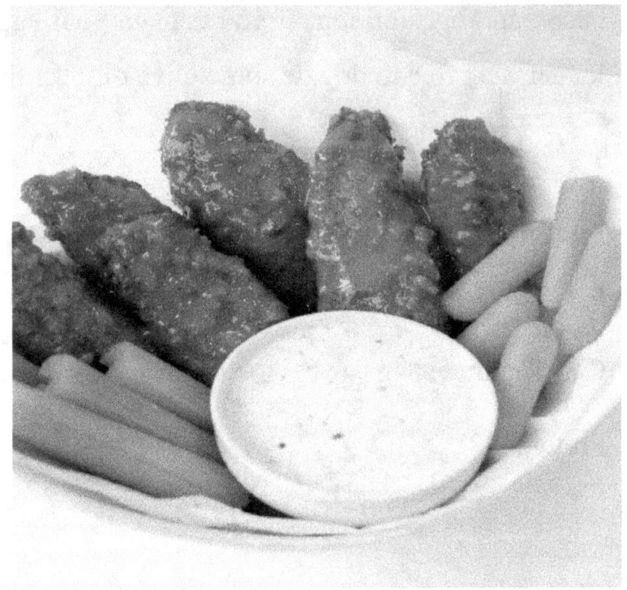

Total Time: 30 minutes

Serves: 4

Ingredients

- 2 cups crushed pork rinds

- 3/4 cup finely grated Parmesan cheese

- 1 teaspoon garlic powder

- 1 teaspoon Italian seasoning

- 1 teaspoon onion powder

- 2 large eggs

- 1 1/2 pounds boneless skinless chicken breasts, cut into

tender-size pieces

- 1 cup buffalo wing sauce

- 1/4 cup butter (1/2 stick)

Instructions

1. Combine the pork rinds, Parmesan cheese, garlic powder, Italian seasoning and onion powder and mix until well incorporated. Pour the mixture into a thin layer on a large plate.

2. Crack the eggs into a shallow bowl and fork whisk. Dip the chicken tenders in the egg wash, and then dredge them in the breading mixture. Make sure both sides are thoroughly coated in the breading mixture.

3. Heat 1 to 2 inches of oil is a high-sided skillet. You can use avocado oil for this. Once the oil is hot and begins to bubble slightly, drop the breaded chicken tenders into the oil. Fry until they are golden brown and crispy on both sides, about 3 minutes each side. Be careful not to flip them too much or else the breading will fall off.

4. Remove the chicken tenders from the oil and place them on paper towels to absorb the excess grease.

5. In a small sauce pan, heat the buffalo wing sauce and the butter over medium heat. Cook until the butter is melted and mixed into the sauce. Transfer the sauce to a large mixing bowl. Toss the tenders in the sauce until

thoroughly coated

Nutrition

- Calories: 335 Kcal

- Fat: 21g

- Carbohydrates: 3g

- Protein: 33g

Air-Fryer Mushrooms Steaks

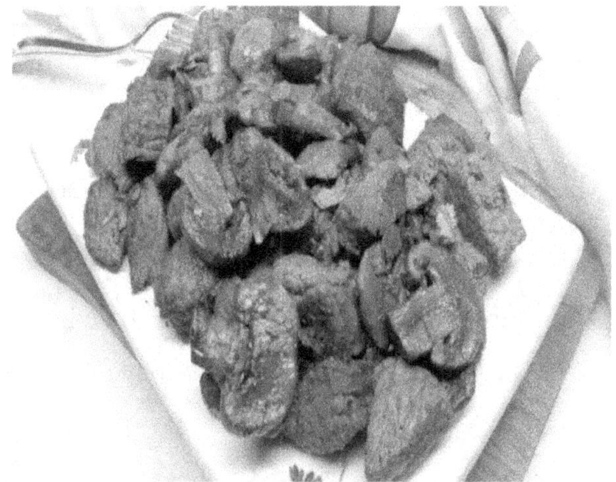

You can make this portobello mushroom steaks that can be cooked in the air fryer or on the grill / barbecue.

Total Time: 15 mins

Servings: 4

Ingredients

- 4 large portobello mushrooms

- 2-3 tbsp olive oil

- 2 tsp tamari soy sauce (or regular soy sauce if not gluten free)

- 1 tsp garlic purée

- salt to taste

Instructions

1. Preheat the Air Fryer to 350F / 180C.

2. Clean the mushrooms with a damp cloth or brush and remove their stems.

3. Mix together the olive oil, tamari soy sauce, garlic purée and salt in a bowl.

4. Add in the mushrooms and mix till coated. You can also use a brush to coat the mushrooms with the mixture. You can cook straight away, or let the mushrooms rest for 10 minutes before cooking.

5. Add the mushrooms to the air fryer basket and cook for 8-10 minutes.

6. Serve the garlic Air Fryer Mushrooms with some salad greens.

Nutrition

- Calories: 84 kcal

- Carbohydrates: 4g

- Protein: 2g

- Fat: 7g

Bratwurst & Vegetables

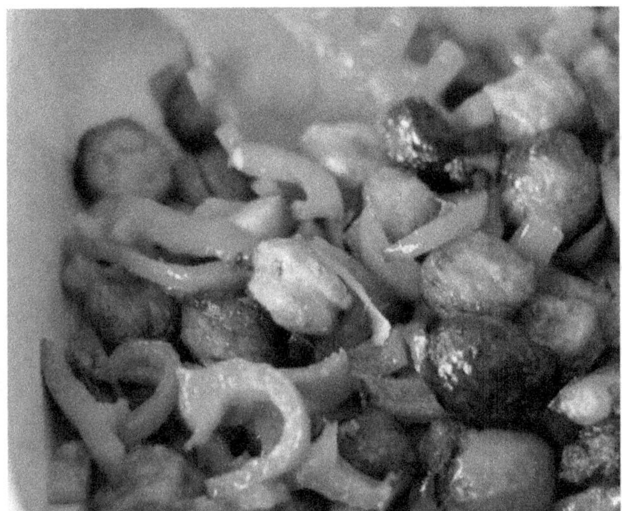

Make a ◻uick, simple meal with this Air Fryer Bratwurst and Vegetables. Perfect for dinner

Yield: 6

Total time: 30 min

Equipment: Airfryer

Ingredients

- 1 Package Bratwurst (4-5 Links)

- 1 Red Bell Pepper, Sliced

- 1 Green Bell Pepper, Sliced

- 1/4 Cup Red Onion, Diced

- 1/2 Tbsp Gluten-Free Cajun Seasoning

Instructions

1. Line the air fryer with foil, if preferred.

2. Add in the vegetables.

3. Sliced the bratwurst into about 1/2 inch size rounds, and then place on top of the vegetables.

4. Evenly sprinkle the Cajun seasoning on top.

5. Air fry at 390 degrees for 10 minutes.

6. Carefully open, stir or mix up.

7. Finish air frying for another 10 minutes.

8. Serve and enjoy!

Nutrition

- Calories: 63 Kcal

- Fat: 4g

- Carbs: 2g

- Protein: 2g

Shawarma Green Beans

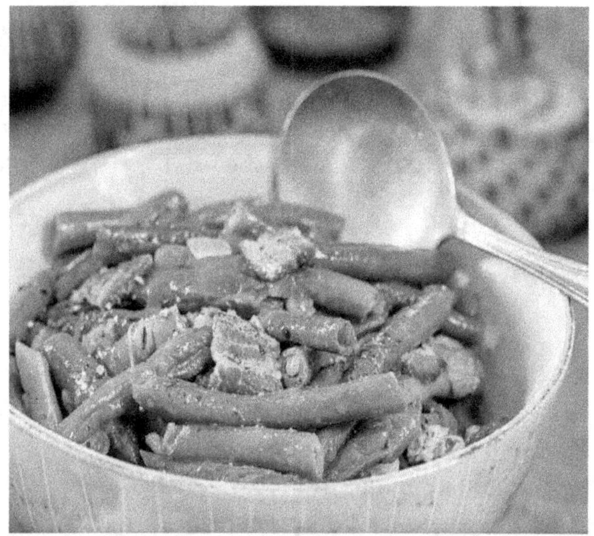

Shawarma Green Beans are a light and flavorful side dish that can be made right in your Air Fryer. They're ready for the table in just 15 minutes from start to finish!

Total Time: 15 minutes

Servings: 2

Equipment: Airfryer

Ingredients

- 2 cups green beans

- 2 tbsp Oil

- 1 tbsp shawarma spice

- 1/2 tsp Salt

Instructions

1. Top and tail the green beans and snap in half, and place in a bowl.

2. Add the oil, shawarma mix and salt and mix well.

3. Place the seasoned green beans in the air fryer basket and set the air fryer for 370ºF for 10 minutes. At the halfway mark, shake the basket and flip over the green beans.

4. Remove and serve.

Nutrition

- Calories: 158 kcal

- Carbohydrates: 8g

- Protein: 2g

- Fat: 14g

Cauliflower Bites

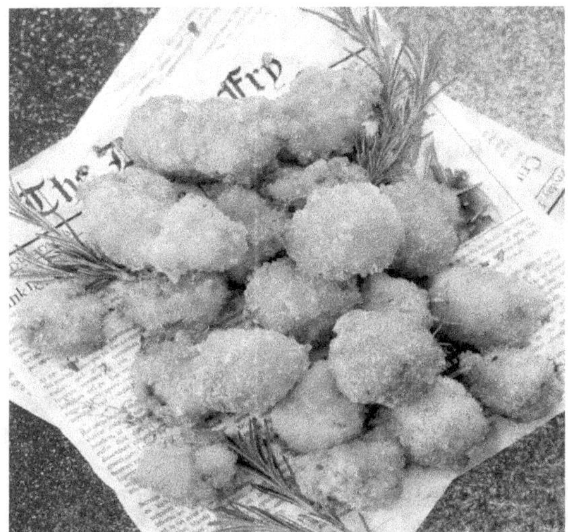

Cauliflower bites are coated in a low carb keto breading. These can be baked, fried or cooked in an air fryer.

Total Time: 35 min

Serves: 4

Equipment: Airfryer

Ingredients

- 12 oz cauliflower, cut into bite sized pieces (about 1/2 a large head of cauliflower)

- cooking oil for frying

- panko bread crumbs

Egg Wash

- 2 large eggs whisked

- 2 tbsp heavy cream

Breading

- 1 cup superfine blanched almond flour

- 1 cup finely grated parmesan cheese, use fresh and not shelf stable kind

- 1 tsp garlic powder

- 1/4 tsp smoked paprika

- 1/4 tsp cayenne pepper, optional if you like a little spice in your breading

Instructions

1. In a small bowl, whisk eggs with heavy cream. Set aside.

2. In a medium bowl, whisk together almond flour, cheese, garlic powder, smoked paprika and cayenne pepper. Set aside.

3. Line a medium baking sheet with parchment paper. Spoon a small amount of breading onto your sheet pan (just enough to cover the bottom of a cauliflower bite).

4. Dip a piece of cauliflower in the egg wash. After it is fully coated, shake it a few times, making sure to shake off any excess egg drippings back into the egg bowl before adding it to the breading. The reason for doing

this is that you don't want the egg drippings going into the breading. The moisture will cause the breading to clump and they will no longer stick to the cauliflower.

5. Place the cauliflower piece onto the small mound of panko bread crumbs, applying a little pressure so those breading sticks to the bottom of the cauliflower.

6. Wipe your hand that was holding the cauliflower so that your hand is also dry before touching the breading. Spoon a small amount of breading over the cauliflower and then use your fingers to press the breading onto the cauliflower until it is fully coated. It is important to keep the breading in a separate bowl, to prevent it from getting wet.

7. Carefully set the cauliflower aside onto a clean part of your baking sheet. Repeat with remaining cauliflower.

8. Spray the basket of your air fryer with cooking oil spray to prevent cauliflower from sticking. Place cauliflower in a single layer into basket, spacing them about 1/2 inch apart. You may need to split the cauliflower in more than one batch. Spray the surface of the cauliflower before closing your air fryer. Coating the outside in oil will help the breading crisp up and brown. Set your air fryer to 375F. Cook for about 12 minutes or until crispy.

Nutrition

- calories: 378 Kcal

- carbohydrates: 7g

- protein: 21g

- fat: 27g

4. DESSERT RECIPES

Chocolate Muffins

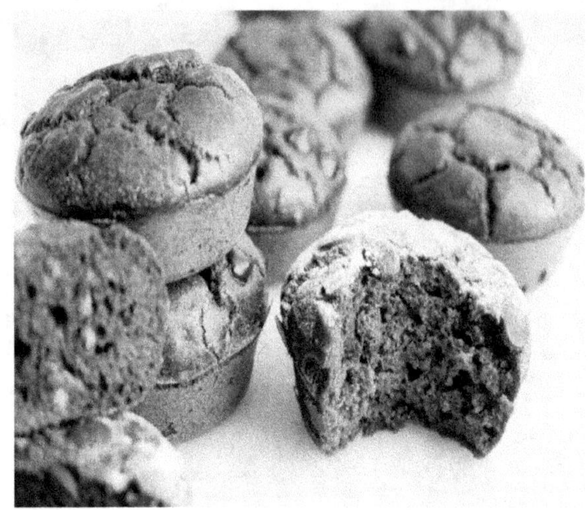

Total Time: 21 minutes

Serves: 6

Ingredients

- 1 cup natural creamy almond butter

- 2/3 cup confectioners erythritol (I use this brand)

- 2 tablespoons unsweetened cocoa powder

- 2 tablespoons peanut butter powder (I use this brand)

- 2 large eggs

- 1 tablespoon melted salted butter, or coconut oil for dairy free

- 2 tablespoons water

- 1 1/2 teaspoons pure vanilla extract

- 1 teaspoon baking soda

- 1/4 cup sugar free dark chocolate baking chips

Instructions

1. Preheat oven to 350°F. Place a silicone mini muffin pan on top of a rimmed baking sheet.

2. In a large mixing bowl, combine the almond butter, erythritol, cocoa powder, peanut butter powder, eggs, butter, water, vanilla extract, and baking soda. Using an elecrtric hand mixer, mix until all ingredients are well combined. It should be a fairly thick dough. Fold in the chocolate chips.

3. Divide the mixture evenly among 18 wells of the mini muffin pan – or 12 regular sized muffins.

4. Bake for 11 minutes. Remove the baking sheet from the oven and place on a cooling rack to allow the muffins to cool before eating.

Nutrition

- Calories: 115Kcal

- Fat: 10g

- Carbohydrates: 3.8g

- Protein: 4g

Mint Chocolate Fudge

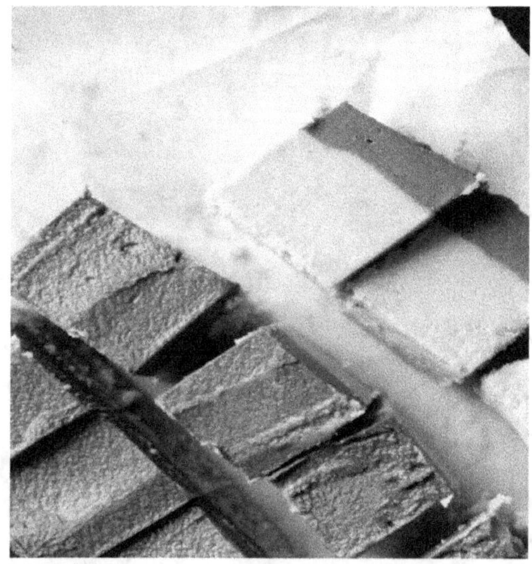

Total Time 8 mins

Ingredients

Mint Cream Layer:

- 2 medium ripe avocados

- 1/2 cup coconut oil at room temp

- 1-2 Tbs cashew butter or almond butter

- 35-45 drops Sweet Leaf vanilla stevia to taste (or 2-3 Tbs powdered coconut sugar)

- 1-2 tsp mint extract to taste

- 2 tsp vanilla

- Dash of pink salt

Additional ingredients for the chocolate layer:

- 1 1/2-2 Tbs cacao to taste

- 1 Tbs cashew butter or almond butter

Instructions

To make the mint layer:

1. Blend all ingredients in a food processor or powerful blender until smooth. (Add the extra Tbs nut butter if you want it more firm.)

2. Scrape down the sides and taste and adjust for sweetness and mint flavor. Blend again.

3. Spread 2/3 of the mint cream into a 5x5" or 6x4" dish lined with parchment paper (save the remaining 1/3 for the top layer)

4. Freeze about 30 minutes until set.

To make the chocolate layer:

1. Add cacao and cashew butter to the leftover mint cream in the food processor and blend smooth. Taste and adjust, adding more cacao, salt or a few more drops of stevia if desired.

2. Spread chocolate over the mint layer and freeze or refrigerate again until set.

3. Slice into 1" s☐uares. Enjoy right away as a silky fudge

bite or freeze for a mini ice cream bar treat!

Nutrition

- Calories: 67 Kcal

- Fats: 7g

- Carbs: 1g

- Protein: 0g

Chocolate Chip Cookies

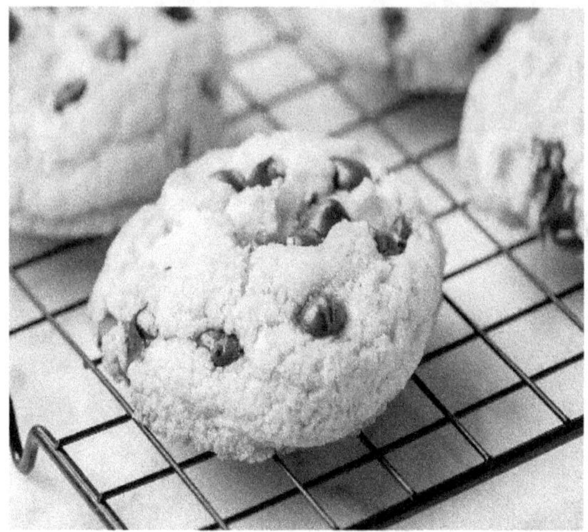

Total Time: 18 minutes

Servings: 10

Ingredients

- 1 cup almond flour

- 1 medium egg

- 2 tbsp double/heavy cream

- 2 tbsp butter unsalted, VERY soft

- 3 tbsp granulated sweetener

- 1 tsp vanilla extract

- 2 oz dark chocolate/chocolate chips (85% minimum or sugar free)

Instructions

1. Preheat the oven to 180 Celsius/356 Fahrenheit

2. Combine all ingredients apart from the chocolate with a fork. Let the dough sit for a few minutes so the flour can absorb the moisture

3. Chop your chocolate and stir into the dough

4. Form dough balls with your hand or spoon the mixture on a baking sheet lined with baking paper. Press down into the desired shape (ca 1/2 cm thick)

5. Bake for ca 13 minutes or until the edges are nicely browned. They are soft when straight out of the oven but firm up as they cool down.

Recipe Notes

1. The mixture makes 10 cookies with a diameter of around 6 cm. Nutrition is calculated per cookie.

2. If you like chewier cookies, make them thicker than 1/2 cm and reduce the baking time to 10 minutes. For crispier cookies, flatten them further.

3. This low carb chocolate chip cookie recipe also works WITHOUT the egg! The end result is crispier (but also more fragile when hot). Add an extra splash of cream to loosen the dough.

Nutrition

- Calories: 132 Kcal

- Fat: 11.2g

- Carbohydrates: 3.6g

- Protein: 2.8g

Pumpkin Snickerdoodle Cookies

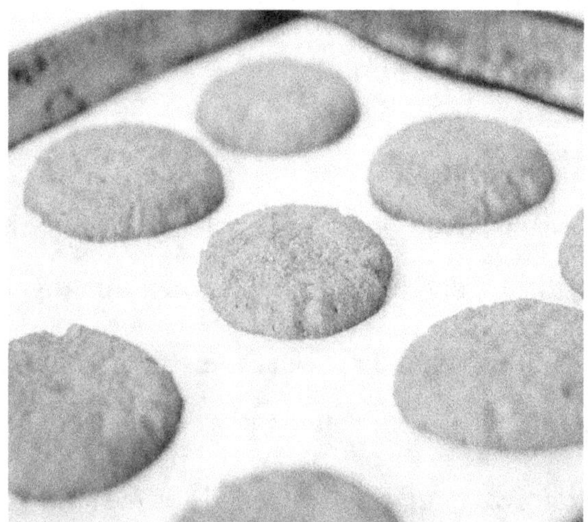

Total Time : 20 min

Serves: 2

Ingredients

The Cookies

- 1 ½ cups almond flour

- ¼ cup salted butter

- ½ cup pumpkin puree

- 1 teaspoon vanilla extract

- ½ teaspoon baking powder

- 1 large egg

- ¼ cup erythritol

- 25 drops liquid stevia

The Topping

- 1 teaspoon pumpkin pie spice

- 2 teaspoons erythritol

Instructions

1. Pre-heat oven to 350°F. Measure out almond flour, erythritol, and baking powder then mix together well.

2. Secondly, measure out the butter, pumpkin puree, vanilla, and li☐uid stevia in a separate container.

3. Microwave mixture if needed for easier mixing. Add all wet ingredients (including the egg) to the almond flour and erythritol.

4. Mix everything together well until a pasty dough is formed.

5. Roll the dough into small balls and set on a cookie sheet covered with a silpat. You should have about 15 cookies in total.

6. Press the balls flat with your hand (or the bottom side of a jar) and bake for 12-13 minutes.

7. While the cookies are cooking, run 2 tsp. erythritol and 1 tsp. pumpkin pie spice through a spice grinder to powder the erythritol.

8. Once the cookies are out of the oven, sprinkle with the topping and let cool completely.

Nutrition

- Calories: 104.53 Kcal

- Fats: 9.4g

- Net Carbs: 1.5g

- Protein: 2.99g

Low Carb Peanut Butter Cookies

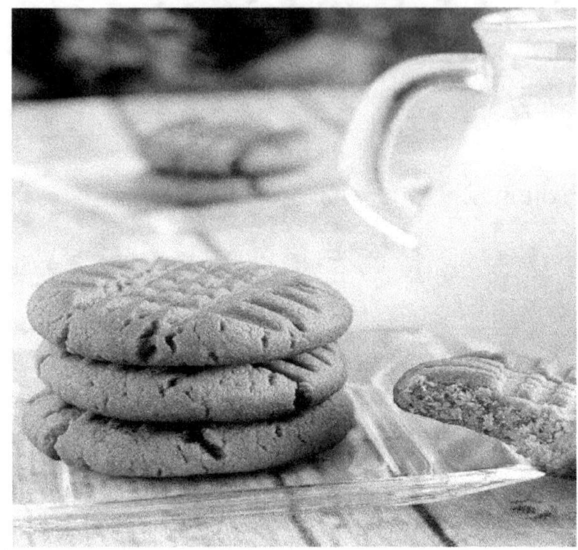

Total Time: 1 hour

Serves: 12

Ingredients

- 1 cup smooth peanut butter (no added sugar)

- 1 large egg

- 2/3 cup erythritol

- 1/2 tsp. baking soda

- 1/2 tsp. vanilla essence

Instructions

1. Preheat oven to 350F (180°C) and line a cookie tray with baking paper. Set aside.

2. Add the erythritol to a Nutribullet or blender and blend until powdered. Set aside.

3. Add all of the ingredients for the peanut butter cookies into a mixing bowl and mix until a smooth dough forms.

4. Measure out 2 tbsp. of the dough and roll between your palms to make round balls and place on your cookie tray. Continue until all the dough has been used.

5. Use a fork to press the cookies down and bake for 12 - 15 minutes depending on your oven. Once they have cooked, remove from the oven and allow to cool for 25 minutes on the cookie tray. Don't touch them yet!

6. Once they have cooled on the cookie tray, transfer the peanut butter cookies to a cooling rack and allow to cool for a further 15 minutes.

Nutrition

- Calories: 140 Kcal

- Fat 10.4g

- Carbohydrates 4g

- Protein 5.8g

CONCLUSION

Intermittent fasting coupled with a keto meal plan is one of the most effective methods we've seen that can improve your overall wellbeing, and is a great tool for weight management.

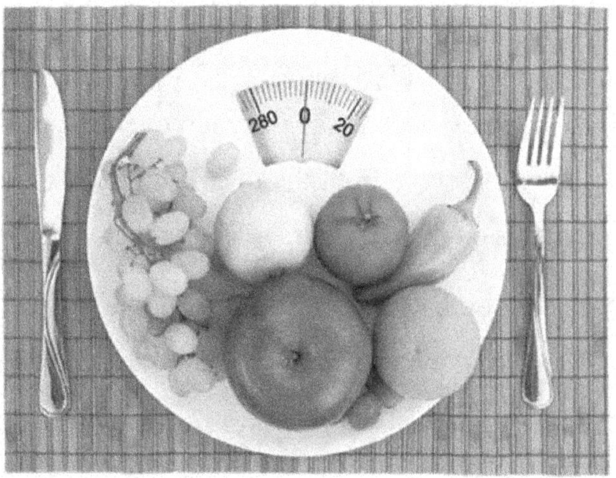

Did you enjoy this book? I would be very pleased if you leave a review on Amazon, and also share your thoughts with me.

www.ingramcontent.com/pod-product-compliance
Lightning Source LLC
Chambersburg PA
CBHW070709250726
48662CB00001B/334